Eusebio Güell Bacigalupi, R. F. Rafael

Immunity through leucomaines

Eusebio Güell Bacigalupi, R. F. Rafael

Immunity through leucomaines

ISBN/EAN: 9783742805775

Manufactured in Europe, USA, Canada, Australia, Japa

Cover: Foto ©Lupo / pixelio.de

Manufactured and distributed by brebook publishing software
(www.brebook.com)

Eusebio Güell Bacigalupi, R. F. Rafael

Immunity through leucomaines

IMMUNITY THROUGH LEUCOMAINES.

BY

EUSEBIO GÜELL BACIGALUPI.

TRANSLATED FROM THE SECOND FRENCH EDITION

BY

R. F. RAFAEL, M.D.

NEW YORK:
J. H. VAIL & CO.,
21 Astor Place.
1889.

CONTENTS.

PART THIRD.

EXPLANATION OF SOME PHENOMENA BY THIS THEORY.

IMMUNITY THROUGH LEUCOMAINES.

The author will be pleased to receive from you an opinion of the merits of this book, which please forward to

J. H. VAIL & CO.,

21 Astor Place, N. Y.,

or to ARTURO CUYÁS,

Kemble Building, N. Y.

INTRODUCTION TO THE FIRST EDITION.

How do vaccines act, and what is their nature ? *

This is what I propose to explain.

Have I disclosed a new law of nature, or merely discov-
·ered a new theory ?

I really believe the former is the case; but as in the code
of these eternal laws there is nothing but absolute truth,
and as we can never be sure of having found it, I enter the
more courageously the vast field of theories where, in the
·existence of doubt, discussion preserves all its rights.

Many ingenious theories exist based on plausible hypotheses; but are they not for the greater part made up of
utopia ?

The one I here present has captivated me as much by
the simplicity and clearness of its reasoning, as on account
of the hopes to which it gives rise for the benefit of mankind, should it be found absolutely true.

If I be mistaken, my readers will, I trust, excuse me;
for is not indulgence indeed previously granted to the
conscientious seeker who has strayed from the right road
guided by data that allured him by their wisdom and
brilliancy ?

---

* Vaccine, from the French *vaccin*, is used here in a general
sense to designate any substance or matter which, being in itself
the product of disease, is introduced into the animal system by inoculation or otherwise, thereby preventing the development of the
same or an analogous distemper in a virulent form.

INTRODUCTION TO THE SECOND EDITION.

For a long number of years, Jenner's discovery had stood as a fact, extraordinary indeed, but isolated and almost unique.

During the last few years, sheep, swine, etc., have been successfully preserved from many diseases by means of inoculations made with substances extracted from the humors engendered by the disease against which protection was sought.

The success of these inoculations directed attention towards mankind, in order to obtain a similar benefit.

Pasteur, with his inoculations against rabies; Ferran, with those against cholera; those made in the West Indies and South America against yellow fever, awoke the interest of savants throughout the world.

It was no longer a question of isolated cases of prophylaxis more or less successful. Every one perceived therein something grander, and felt that a new method was rising to the view of the scientific world.

But if it was indeed a method, what was the principle that this method obeyed unconsciously?

Mr. Pasteur, who had for a number of years dedicated his attention to these labors, and who had endeavored to discover this principle, proceeded rightly and went to the bottom of the question on referring to the same cause the effect produced by inoculations, and the fact presented by nature of the non-recurrence of infectious diseases. This point of view was of the highest importance, and offered a much vaster field to observers.

Several theories were invented to explain these phenomena, the most important of which have been already mentioned in the first edition of the present work.

M. Pasteur gave two or three explanations, but he doubted, and, consequently, did not dare to decide definitely. This great experimenter, to whom science is indebted for so many and such important discoveries, and who, by this means, had covered his name with glory, hardly dared to soar in the region of theories. When he conceived one, he immediately rejected it if he failed to find a direct proof of it in new experiments.

M. Chauveau, who, likewise, had studied these questions deeply, directed his observations so as to find an explanation for the phenomena of immunity.

His observations have, in my opinion, a very great importance, and his interpretation of several experimental facts and some natural phenomena will always stand as sure guides on the road that the theory of immunity must follow.

At the time when science was at about this height, I found an explanation that comprised both the phenomena of infectious diseases and the experimental facts of vaccination; not, indeed, by any new discovery, nor by a new substance before unknown, but by the application of a law known to all, but which nevertheless remained barren for science. This generality struck and captivated me, for universality is a condition of natural laws.

Starting, then, from this height, I descended towards the phenomena presented by infectious diseases and vaccinations.

Thinking that others had harmed the cause of the principle by attaching too great an importance to experimental facts, I abandoned this ground completely, and sought an aid from reasoning and logic.

It is thus I arrived at conclusions that some have thought too daring. I believed, nevertheless, that sooner or later they would render a service to science. Many savants have likewise so thought who have referred to my work either in scientific reviews or in Academies.

Among these, some have found, by means of the theory of Immunity through Leucomaines, an explanation of phenomena hitherto unaccounted for. Some of these explanations add so great a value to this theory, and are in themselves of such great interest, that I transcribe them in this edition as a continuation of the part of my work dedicated to the "Explanation of Several Phenomena."*

Others have encouraged investigators to follow this new road in the belief that it may lead to a true knowledge of pathogeny. How far this advice has been followed I know not, but I find two notes presented this year to the Academy of Sciences, the names of the authors of which, and the importance of the facts therein related, have a decisive force in favor of my theory.†

In September, 1886, I published the first edition of the work, "Immunity through Leucomaines."

* Part Third, Chapter IV.
† See Appendix, Notes III. and IV.

Two years have since elapsed. During this time a great number of works have appeared bearing on these matters; for light is constantly growing in this new science.

Has there been any scientific work of a similar nature that destroys the reasonings I have made?

Many studies there are that attribute immunity to other very different causes, but there are also two or three very important ones that are a corrroboration of my work.

In the month of February, 1887, M. Pasteur sent to the annals of the institute that bears his name a letter, the second part of which was dedicated to the theory of immunity.

About this same time (May, 1887,) M. Chauveau published in the *Revue de Médécine* a study also on immunity. These two studies are entirely in accord with my theory, which receives thereby a new sanction.*

My work has not failed to meet with objections, but these are in fact very few in number. Moreover, I do not believe that their force is enough to harm the development I have given to my theory. I invite the attention of the reader to the chapter in which I discuss the value of these objections.

* See Appendix, Notes I. and II.

PART FIRST.

THEORY OF IMMUNITY.

PART FIRST.

THEORY OF IMMUNITY.

CHAPTER I.

There are but few remedies in medicine whose action is positive and certain, and among these, vaccination holds the first place.

In small-pox, fowl-cholera, murrain, the rot, peripneumonia, and other diseases among animals, and more recently in the cure of rabies, the action of the curative and preservative medicament produces an effect of striking infallibility.

It is therefore of the highest importance to find out the common cause of such an extensive action, and it must be admitted that there is something similar in the manner of acting of all these vaccines.

I well know that the prophylactic action of the vaccines has been called upon to explain their effect, but I cannot believe in the exactness of the theories invented for this purpose, as they have been proved false by the latest experiments of M. Pasteur and other savants, in inoculations recently practised.

Two questions thus present themselves: What is vaccine?* How does it act?

When no other vaccine was known but that for small-pox, taken from a cow having a disease similar in symptoms and effects, it was thought that the introduction of the virus in the body of man, producing a slight distemper similar to small-pox, rendered his nature refractory to the greater disorder.

And still, there was another way of being vaccinated, viz., by acquiring the disease itself; as it is well known that those who have had the small-pox have an immunity from the disease for a longer or shorter period of time.

Afterwards, when veterinary art had made greater progress, vaccinations were practised by extracting the virus from the disease itself;† it was therefore not a similar, but the actual disease in a mild form that was sought to be produced in the individual vaccinated; this being a nearer approach to the natural vaccination produced by the sickness itself.

We were thus led to believe that it was the malady in itself, although under a mild form, that gave rise to the immunity.

* In order to be more clear and brief in my explanations, I will use the words *vaccine* and *vaccination* in the general sense of any virus and the fact of its inoculation with the purpose of producing immunity.

† "Not long ago, under the influence of M. Pasteur, but little faith was placed in artificial immunity, unless produced by the efficacy of inoculations made with races of virus attenuated by successive breeding or culture, thus ignoring the excellent results daily obtained by other practitioners who employed only the strongest virus." (*Grenoble Congress*, 1885. Paper by M. CHAUVEAU.)

But, as M. Chauveau well set forth in his paper read at
the Congress of Grenoble in August, 1885,* there are many
vaccinations among beasts which present no symptoms of
the disease, and which would therefore perhaps make us
believe that the disease had not been produced from which
immunity was sought.

By accepting the theory that it was the disease itself,
stronger or weaker, that was produced in the vaccinated
individual, the action was very plausibly explained.

It was said that, in the first place, the inoculated matter
contained a virus attenuated by different cultures or by its
natural conditions as that of cows for small-pox.

This virus, which according to the studies of the most

---

*Other persons make the contrary objection, averring that no
account is to be taken of such inoculations, as they are inactive
and in no case produce anything resembling the symptoms of
cholera.

It is now easier to answer this objection than formerly, owing
to the repeated number of analogous instances. Vaccine virus in-
serted in the connective tissue of an individual of the bovine species does not produce any of the cutaneous manifestations characteristic of cow-pox; and nevertheless the immunity of animals
thus inoculated is so great that it is impossible thereafter to produce the vaccinal exanthem by sub-epidemic prickings. The intra-
venous injections of the same vaccine virus in the equine species
but rarely gives rise to this exanthem; and still, the animals not
having this symptom are as well preserved as the others from the
effects of the classical cutaneous inoculation. Again, the intra-
venous injection in an ox of the emphysematous virus of anthrax
or the peripneumonic virus, etc., produce neither Chabert's disease nor peripneumonia, nor anything that resembles these maladies in their symptoms; but nevertheless they give a very solid
immunity. Similar results are obtained with the subcutaneous
injections of the peripneumonic virus. (Grenoble Congress, *Le
Temps*, 16th August, 1885.)

competent men, is a living being, a *microbe** of animal or
vegetable nature, takes from the human economy the elements necessary for its existence, and on absorbing these
substances, it renders the system refractory to the life and
growth of a similar microbe when presenting itself to produce the disease.

Even admitting the existence of attenuated microbes, it
would always be necessary for those introduced by vaccination into man to multiply and reach the same result as the
microbes of the disease, in order to absorb all the substances
favorable to their nourishment. To attain this end, the
very fact of their being weaker will oblige us to admit that
they are more numerous, and in this case the same fatal
consequences should be feared as from the disease; as instead of the morbid power of each microbe we would have
that of a much larger number.‡

---

* The expression *microbe*, taken from the French, meaning in
fact simply *small living being*, implies nothing as to the animal or
vegetable nature of the beings here treated on. It has been
adopted by M. Pasteur and approved by M. Littré, whose com-
petency in terminology is universally recognized. It has come
into general use in France within the last four or five years,
and can now be considered as definitely acquired to the French
language. (*Les Microbes, les ferments et les moisissures*, by Dr. E.
L. Trouessart. Introd. p. 4.)

† M. Béchamp calls the microbes *microzymæ*, or small ferments,
as the chemical reactions resulting from their vital activity are
generally fermentations.

‡ But this theory is not free from certain objections. Grawitz
says it requires to be explained how the economy which can provide sustenance for the enormous proliferation of the microbes of
a dangerous virulent disease, such as malignant rot or anthrax, can
be exhausted by the much more moderate vegetation of the same

Finding all these explanations very unlikely, I happened to read in an article of Doctor Respaut* that M. Ferran did not employ the microbe for his vaccinations, and that the fact of immunity was produced by the broth into which the microbes had been introduced and bred.

In another note published this winter, M. Ferran himself asserted that it was by habituating the nature of man to the poison produced by the microbe † that he rendered it refractory to the disease, just the same as immunity from the fatal effects of morphia is obtained by its frequent use.

Here we have a totally different explanation, according to which, death is not caused by the microbe, but by the poison it produces, and to this same poison is attributed the medical action.

This change in the effects of a substance that passes from the toxic to the prophylactic state is not explained, and M. Ferran says: "Whoever will explain this will also explain the effects of my vaccination."

It appears to me contrary to human reason to attribute life and death to the same cause.

If in the disease the poison is the cause of death, it is difficult to admit that by introducing it into the body we pre-

virus when attenuated. (*Les Immunités morbides*, by Dr. W. Du-BREUILH, p. 190.)

* Journal *Le Temps*, issue of 23d July, 1885.

† As the disease of cholera is the effect of an intoxication by a poisonous fungus, *comma bacillus*, immunity from it is explained by a phenomenon of tolerance of the organism for this poison. The inoculated microbe is not propagated throughout, and not at all in the cellular tissue, there being therefore no danger in employing it for vaccination. The action of such vaccination is due to the active substance formed by the inoculated germs within their protoplasm.—(M. J. FERRAN. Letter to M. Charles Cameron.)

vent its further action when produced by the disease; because there would be an addition of poisons, and the addition of two homogeneous quantities must always give a larger one, and consequently in this case the poison would be more powerful.

It was on reading these notes of M. Ferran, translated by M. Respaut, that I conceived another explanation much simpler, which demonstrates in a much more logical manner all phenomena relating to infectious diseases and to their vaccines.

The exposition of the theory derived therefrom will be the object of the present work.

CHAPTER II.

That the reader may better understand our theory on cholera vaccine, and on all vaccines of the infections maladies in general, I will lead him through the same path of reasoning by which I myself have reached my present convictions.

The starting point was the following observation taken from a note of M. Ferran:

"The microbe does not reproduce in the cellular tissue, and its prophylactic action is due to a sort of accustoming or habituation of the organism to the active diffusible substance generated by the microbe."

In this case it is not the microbe more or less attenuated of the disease, or of a similar disease, that produces by inoculation immunity. According to M. Ferran, it is the broth containing the active diffusible substance already generated by the microbe that has this effect.

Moreover, we know from Virchow that the existence of the comma bacillus as the specific micro-organism of Asiatic cholera is now placed beyond a doubt.

And for my part, I also believe that we must accept with Van Ermengen, basing himself on Koch's conclusions, "that in the absence of any other contagious matter of an animated nature, except the bacilli, these must be admitted as the agents of transmission and the cause itself of the disease."

We have. therefore, two distinct facts: on one side the existence of the micro-organisms, *comma bacilli*, as the cause of the disease of cholera,* and on the other, the fact ascertained by M. Ferran that the introduction into the system of a quantity of broth that has served for breeding these same comma bacilli produces immunity.†

What is then the composition of this broth that produces such a benefit?

If it acts as a poison, what does it act on?

* The third and last hypothesis is that there exists a relation of cause to effect between the choleric processus and the comma bacilli. For me, the fact is fully proved. (KOCH.)

After this examination of numerous bacteria, which, each in turn, without much appearance of reason, have been declared identical to those of cholera, I believe I am justified in concluding that till now nothing has been found at all like that of Koch elsewhere than among subjects attacked by cholera. (DR. E. VAN ERMENGEN.)

Others have asked, "With what do you practise these inoculations? Is it with the cultures of comma bacilli? Are you sure that this microbe is the essential agent of cholera?"

This is a serious objection, but it loses ground every day. (French Association for the advancement of Science—Grenoble Congress—*Le Temps*, 6th August, 1885.)

In my belief, these organisms are the cause of cholera, and precede it. Some think they are the effect of the malady; but as I have already said, this is impossible. (DR. KOCH, Imperial Council of Berlin; sitting of 26th July, 1884.)

† I well know that many readers will reject this hypothesis, asserting that the efficacy of M. Ferran's system has not been proved; but I pray the reader to follow my reasoning, even supposing my premises false; for in all scientific researches, purely imaginary suppositions are sometimes allowed, when having for their object the discovery of either a law or a theory. (THE AUTHOR.)

These are the questions we are about to examine.

The name of microbe is given to any living being too small to be visible to the naked eye.

The comma bacillus * here mentioned is a living being, either vegetable or animal; it matters not which for the point of view under which I study the question.

What is the necessary condition for the life of every living being? The condition *sine qua non* is that it be in a medium favorable to its life, that it assimilate the substances in this medium, and after transforming them eliminate them, that is to say, give back other substances.

Let us now examine what under this relation occurs in the case of more perfected beings, whose functions are better known to us.

If a man be placed in an apartment previously provided with different kinds of food, and the apartment be hermetically closed, this man, after the lapse of a certain length of time, will become ill, his breathing will be more and more difficult, and death will in a short time supervene.

The reason is that the air within the apartment will have been totally changed; the oxygen has become more and

* The comma bacillus, as well as every other organism, must follow the laws of vegetation, like all larger plants. It must reproduce itself, generating its like; and it cannot come from a vegetable of another kind, and much less can it be the product of nothing. (DR. KOCH; sitting of July 26th, 1884; Imperial Council of Berlin.)

more scarce, and been replaced by vapor of water, carbonic acid, and the ammoniacal gases produced by the secretions and excretions of the subject.

Sooner or later, the change within this space will be complete. All the elements necessary to the life of man will have been replaced by other elements either useless or injurious.

If for our experiment we take a vegetable, the result will be similar.

If a plant in a pot filled with earth be placed under a glass globe, it will have all the elements necessary to its life, but in a limited degree and in a restricted space, thus enabling us to collect the products of its existence.

Before long the leaves will dry up, the color will fade, and the plant will irretrievably die.

The beneficent influence of the sun that excites the activity of the globules of chlorophyllum placed in the cavities of the cellulose will soon become powerless, there being no more carbon to absorb. Oxygen in the gaseous state will be contrary to its life. The water will disappear on account of the partial reduction it undergoes in the interior of the plants; the earth will lose its ammonia, its potash, phosphoric acid, etc. All the elements necessary to vegetable life will disappear and be replaced by elements noxious to such a life.

A fish in a glass globe, even when left in contact with the air, will perish within a few days if the products of its life are left in the water.

In all living beings, the products of life are noxious to this same life.

Therefore, the broth used for breeding or culture by M.

Ferran must contain, either in suspension or solution, substances intoxicating to the comma bacilli.*

From what we have previously said it is evident that, if in this broth new microbes be introduced, they will perish there, just as a man would die on entering an apartment where others have already died after having absorbed all the elements of life existing therein and leaving there the products of their own existence.

M. Ferran's system consists, therefore, in introducing into the human organism the leucomaines † of the comma bacilli, and if the system has in reality any efficacy, it is because, when these bacilli enter the organism through contagion, the presence of their own leucomaines renders their life feeble and finally causes their death.

By another reasoning, we can likewise sustain the same thesis.

* The comma bacillus, like any other organism, must follow the laws of vegetation the same as large plants. (Dr. Koch, sitting of 26th July, 1884, Imperial Council of Berlin.)

† At present, the expression *ptomaines*, which means any cadaverical base, is used indifferently to designate the organic bases extracted from the albuminoid matters undergoing putrefaction, or those which can be extracted from the tissues of living men and beasts, and which are produced during the normal state of life; on account of their double origin, I propose to give to these bases the name of *leucomaines* from $\lambda\varepsilon\acute{u}\varkappa\omega\mu\alpha$ (white of eggs). (*Dictionary of pure and applied Chemistry* by A. D. Wurtz.)

Note.—In using throughout this work the word *leucomaines*, I will not give it the restricted sense of Wurtz, but shall intend to designate by it the totality or a part of the products of elimination which are the result of the vital functions of any micro-organism whatever. (The Author.)

According to what we have already said, we have two men vaccinated against cholera in two different ways, one by having had the disease, and the other by introducing into his system the leucomaines of the comma bacillus.

In all probability, if we find anything common in these two individuals, this point in common will be the cause of their immunity.

Since M. Ferran tells us that his broth contains no other active substance producing immunity except the poison eliminated by the microbes, we must see if we can find this substance in the man whose state of immunity is subsequent to the disease.

The microbe propagating throughout the system takes therefrom all the substances necessary for its nutrition.*

These substances are likewise necessary to the vital functions of man.

Man, like every other organized being, requires the ele-

---

* By the acts of its nutrition, the microbe occasions the gravity of the disease and causes death. This is easy to be understood. The microbe, for instance, is *aerobic*, absorbing during its existence large quantities of oxygen and burning up a great number of principles of the medium in which it is bred. This can be easily proved by comparing the extracts of the chicken broth before and after the cultivation of the small organism. Everything tends to show that this oxygen, necessary to its life, is taken from the blood globules and absorbed through the vessels, and the proof is that during life, and even frequently long before the approach of death, the crest of diseased fowls is seen to take a violaceous tint, while yet the microbes have either not entered the blood or entered in quantities so small as to elude microscopical investigation. (PASTEUR, *Comptes rendus*, Academy of Sciences, 3d May, 1880.)

ments which constitute the aggregate whole of his system
in determined quantities and proportions, this quantity and
proportion constituting the state of health.

The loss of a larger or smaller quantity of these elements
alters the equilibrium, and the disturbance that arises thereby is what we term disease.

Now, if we represent the state of health by the formula
$3a+3b+3c+3d$, that of sickness or disease will be repre-
sented by $1a+1b+1c+1d$.

Man after illness and convalescence enjoys perfect health
which proves that he has regained all the substances previously lost, i. e., he has returned to the first formula $3a+3b+3c+3d$.

But with these substances and this formula he did not
have immunity before his sickness.

Therefore, this formula does not bestow immunity. And
still, this immunity exists after an infectious disease; consequently this condition must be attributed to the presence
of new substances.

The formula representing this state would thus be $3a+3b+3c+3d+x$.

M. Chauveau has made a very important observation
that upholds what we have just said.*

* "In the note stating the facts with which I have just dealt,
M. Pasteur discusses again (*Comptes rendus*, page 536) the interpretation that should be given to the immunity acquired or
strengthened by a first inoculation. Although my name has been
mixed up with this discussion, I would have taken no part in it,
had it not appeared to me that M. Pasteur has not well understood
my idea and intentions. I have not pretended to erect a new theory regarding immunity (the moment for it not appearing to me
as yet come), and to oppose this theory to that of M. Pasteur.

Let us then search for the substance x of the formula that represents the state of immunity co-existent with a state of perfect health.

The disease-producing microbes during their life within

During the course of my observations, I came across a fact to which it was difficult to apply, as I thought, the theory adopted by M. Pasteur, and so I mentioned it. This difficulty still exists. I was making a comparative study of inoculations practised with very small quantities of infectious agents and those in which a large quantity is employed, both on Algerian sheep endowed only with their natural immunity, and on other sheep in which immunity has been strengthened by one or several inoculations. I have shown (and I have the means of rendering my demonstration more complete) that the chances of being able to produce rot completely, that is to say fatally, are far greater when inoculating at one time a large number of infectious agents. Now, how can this fact be made to agree with the theory of exhaustion?

"How can a system from which *one or several precious cultures have absorbed the greater part of the matters necessary to the proliferation of the infectious agents of anthrax be a better field for the increase of these agents when sown abundantly than when introduced in quantities reduced to the minimum? If the poor nature of the ground is an obstacle to the culture, would not this barrenness manifest itself more evidently in proportion to the germs sown?* Would not the same fact that happens in a culture-tube manifest itself in the animal system? This is my objection. I have stated it in a theoretical interpretation of the fact I had observed, by saying that the *comparative bacteridian inoculations with small or large quantities of virus acted as if in the organism of the animal there existed matters or other agents against which the infectious agents had to struggle in order to live and multiply, and over which they triumphed the more easily when introduced in larger quantities.*

"It is with the greatest pleasure that I will see this objection cleared from the theory adopted by M. Pasteur—a theory based on facts brought to light by a very captivating experiment to which I have not denied the testimony of my admiration." (Note of M. CHAUVEAU, *Academy of Sciences*, 18th October, 1880.)

the animal system, and while fulfilling their vital functions, must necessarily leave therein the products resulting from their existence.

These substances will remain in the individual for a longer or shorter space of time after the disappearance of the distemper. They are the same as those contained in the broth used for breeding which we have before mentioned.

Therefore these substances which we call *leucomaines*, and which are to be found both in a man enjoying immunity after a sickness and in one in whom it is due to M. Ferran's vaccination, are in reality those which produce the benefit of immunity.

By still a third process of reasoning, we will reach the same conclusions.

Infectious diseases are produced by micro-organisms. These disorders present the character of non-recurrence (*non-recidive*).

The state of immunity following the diseases must be either the effect of the abstraction by the microbes of substances already existing in the animal system, or else due to the presence of new substances.

The former of these two theses must be rejected after the observation made by M. Chauveau, and we must therefore accept the fact that it is the presence of some substance that produces immunity.

As the state of immunity is always subsequent to the presence in the animal system of micro-organisms, it must be admitted that the substance producing this immunity has been degenerated by these micro-organisms.

Why should the substance produced by the micro-organism, which has been the cause of disease, give immunity against such disease?

This is the result of a general law.

As has already been stated, in all living beings the substances produced and eliminated by their vital functions are poisonous to their own life.*

The leucomaines of micro-organisms must therefore be opposed to their vitality.†

* One of the most interesting facts observed in the growth of septic micro-organisms is this, that the products of the decomposition started and maintained by them have a most detrimental influence on themselves, inhibiting their power of multiplication, in fact, after a certain amount of these products has accumulated, the organisms become arrested in their growth, and finally may be altogether killed. Thus the substances belonging to the aromatic series, indol, skatol, phenol, and others which are produced in the course of putrefaction of proteids, have a most detrimental influence on the life of many micro-organisms, as has been shown by Wernich and others. (Dr. E. KLEIN, *Micro-organisms and Disease,* p. 235.)

Urea is the last residue of the combustion of the nitrogenous substances and is eliminated through the urine.

The cessation of the expulsion of this urea gives rise to a disease which is the effect of the intoxication produced by the diffusion of this substance in the blood.

It is therefore a substance that must be eliminated, and which, when retained within the system, manifests its poisonous properties. (THE AUTHOR.)

† But is this in reality the only explanation possible of the phenomena? Strictly speaking, no. The fact of non-recurrence can be explained by admitting that the life of the microbe, instead of taking away or destroying certain matters in the bodies of animals, adds new ones which are an obstacle to the further growth

Consequently the immunity produced must be attributed

of the microbe. The history of the life of the lower beings above all others authorizes such a supposition. The excretions arising from vital functions may be opposed to the performance of functions of the same nature. During certain fermentations, antiseptical products are observed to be generated by the act of fermentation itself which put an end to the active life of the ferments and to the fermentations long before these are completed. In the cultures of microbes, there might be a formation of products, the presence of which would in reality be sufficient to explain non-recurrence and protection. (PASTEUR, *Comptes rendus*, Academy of Sciences, 26th April, 1880.)

Many microbes seem to give rise during their breeding to substances having the property of being harmful to their own growth. (*Comptes rendus, Academy of Sciences*, 26th October, 1885. *Note* by PASTEUR.)

When the microbe acquires a certain age in the liquid, has exhausted therefrom all the substances capable of being assimilated and voided in its own products of elimination, of which it not only has no need, but must by all means avoid the presence of, we can observe the formation at one or several points of the filament, or at one of the extremities of the short and isolated joint, a small mass more refractive and brilliant than the rest of the protoplasm, and whose outline, at no time very distinct, grows blacker and thicker. This is the spore. (*Le Microbe et la Maladie* by E. DU-CLAUX, p. 30.)

Frequently it is sufficient for the bacteria to have lived for a certain length of time in a medium in order to render this medium unfit for their vegetation, on account of the accumulation in too large quantities of products of decomposition detrimental to their growth. It is thus that *lactic fermentation is arrested after a short time through the formation of lactic acid.* For the fermentation to continue, it is necessary to add a sufficient quantity of chalk or white zinc to neutralize the acid as it goes forming. (*Lessons on bacteria*, by M. DE BARY. Translated with notes by M. WASSER-ZUG, p. 106.)

In other species, particularly in those with endospores, it could be said that the spores are not formed until the substratum neces-

to the intoxicating action of the leucomaines on the micro-organisms that give rise to the disease.

sary to the vegetation of the species has become exhausted, or in other words, until it becomes unfit for this vegetation. We might ask whether the explanation of this phenomenon is to be sought for in the fact of the total consumption of all the useful nutritive elements, or *because there has been an accumulation of the products of elimination*, or else because, etc. (*Lessons on bacteria*, by M. DE BARY. Translated by M. WASSERZUG, p. 109.)

M. Duclaux, on treating of the culture of the *aspergillus niger* in the nutritive medium composed by M. Raulin, says: "The introduction of one gramme of iron into the nourishing medium produces an increase of over 800 grammes in the crop. Notwithstanding this resemblance, the manner of working of the zinc is entirely different from that of the iron. The zinc enters the plant as a constituent element of its tissues; the only use for the iron is its action in destroying as soon as formed a poison secreted by the plant, and which, if allowed to accumulate in the liquid, would finally kill the plant. This poison is one of those excretions that all living beings produce, and which they must at any cost rid themselves of." (*Le Microbe et la Maladie*, by E. DUCLAUX, p. 69.)

" According to M. Toussaint the microbes deposit in the blood of animals, where they multiply, a matter that may become a vaccine to them. By filtering in cold in one case, and in the other by raising the temperature of the liquid to 55° C. (131° F.), the bacteria are either separated or killed. The inoculation of blood thus filtered or heated would introduce into the bodies of inoculated animals the vaccinal matter deprived of bacteria. Moreover, M. Toussaint arbitrarily added to his explanations his belief in a pretended phlogogenous action of carbuncular blood. If his exposition of facts had any foundation, the question of the preservative action of virus as I have presented it would have to be all gone over again."

These observations are contained in a note read by M. Pasteur to the Academy of Sciences, in which he undertakes to prove that the interpretation given by M. Toussaint is inadmissible. When the reading of this communication was finished, M. Bouley declared that M. Toussaint had later on acknowledged that his interpretation was erroneous. And now, after the lapse of six years, M. Pasteur is no longer sure of his first theory; for in a note addressed lately to the Academy on the question of vaccine for rabies, he is disposed to revise experiments he had made, guided by a supposition similar to that of M. Toussaint, which had also occurred to him in his observations of the phenomena accompanying the vaccination against fowl-cholera. (THE AUTHOR.)

While all bacteria are capable of disintegrating organic combinations containing nitrogen, they in their turn help to produce certain chemical products which in some cases are definite for a definite species. Such is the case with the various bacteria connected with the fermentations producing lactic acid, butyric acid, and acids belonging to the aromatic series. On many bacteria connected with putrefaction, and also on some pathogenic organisms, these chemical products have a deleterious effect. Small quantities impede their growth, and sufficiently large quantities kill them altogether. (*Micro-organisms and Disease*, by DR. E. KLEIN, page 55.)

CHAPTER III.

1st. All infectious diseases are the result of the disturbance arising in the animal organism from the loss of substances necessary to its economy, that disappear by being absorbed during the acts of nutrition of numerous microorganisms.

2d. The state of immunity, of a longer or shorter duration, in an individual having previously suffered from an infectious disease, is not the effect of a negative condition of his economy; that is to say, it is not because his organism has been deprived of the substances necessary to the life of the microbe, but rather because the leucomaines of this latter are there present; and this state of immunity will last just as long as these leucomaines remain there.

3d. Vaccination, to preserve from an infectious distemper, should therefore consist in introducing into the organism by artificial means the leucomaines of the microbe that produces the disease against which protection is sought.

4th. The production of these leucomaines may be obtained either by means of what till now has been termed a culture, or by introducing the microbe in a medium of the animal system where it cannot propagate, but yet may prolong its existence sufficiently to allow it to produce the quantity of leucomaines necessary to insure immunity.*

* It was not remembered that it is necessary to bear in mind not only the quality of the virus, but likewise the manner in which it is put in contact with the animal economy. Now, to judge *a priori* the work of M. Ferran, if there has in reality been any such, it is absolutely necessary to be perfectly familiarized with the fol lowing principle, established chiefly by the labors of the Lyons school, viz.: that the *channel* of introduction of any virus can exert a considerable influence on its effects.

Let us develop and demonstrate this proposition.

Some kinds of virus, like that of glanders, rot, etc., always manifest their effects with the same energy on those animals that are endowed with the greatest receptivity, whatever the channel through which they enter the animal economy.

Whether they be deposited in the digestive tube, the circulatory current, the deep layers of the epidermis, or the subcutaneous connective tissue, they always produce glanders or malignant rot, generally fatal.

But this indifference of virus as regards the channel of introduction is not a general fact. With vaccine or cow-pox virus entirely different phenomena take place, as has been shown by the studies of M. Chauveau.

In animals of the bovine species, superficial cutaneous inoculation will produce the characteristic pustules; but the subcutaneous injection never will, developing only in this case a larger or smaller tumor of the connective tissue. In both cases the animals are perfectly vaccinated, because further cutaneous inoculations produce no effect. Finally, if the virus be injected into the blood-current, no effect whatever will be produced, and the action on the animal will be void—so much so that, if reinoculated sub-epi-dermically, the point of injection will be the seat of splendid vaccinal pustules.

In the equine species, the virus acts in the same manner, with this only difference (the demonstration of which has been very important as regards the theory of immunity), viz.: that the intervascular injections are not inactive as in oxen. Sometimes, though seldom, the activity of the virus is manifested by the presentation

5th. If during a state of immunity produced by an infectious distemper the individual enjoys perfect health, it must be inferred from this fact that the leucomaines of the micro-organisms that have caused the disease are perfectly compatible with the state of health, and consequently vaccination produced by the direct introduction of the leucomaines should not in this case occasion intoxicating symptoms.

6th. Only in the case of vaccination being made with the microbe itself can the presence of morbid symptoms be accepted.*

of a vaccinal exanthem more or less similar to that of the natural disease.

At other times, and this happens the most frequently, no local or general sign of disease is observed, except a very light and passing elevation of temperature; but the injection produces on each and every subject, without exception, vaccinal immunity, so that it is no longer possible to make vaccine pustules appear on the skin by sub-epidermic prickings.

M. Chauveau calls particular attention to this last point, that when immunity against a disease is desired to be created, *it is not necessary to produce the disease nor an aggregate of symptoms more or less attenuated.*

The attenuation of the effects may be carried so far as to render it absolutely impossible to recognize the disease, so much so that it may be said that there has been no disease whatever; and nevertheless, the immunity determined by this sort of artificial distemper is none the less sure. (Greenoble Congress, *Le Temps*, 16th August, 1885.)

* If a parcel of guinea-pigs be injected with just half the quantity that would be fatal, they acquire an immunity that renders them capable of resisting doses that before would infallibly have killed them. To prove this fact we need but to take two sets of guinea-pigs of the same age, one of which sets has been previously endowed with immunity by means of injection. If into the individuals of these two sets mortal doses be injected, those previously

cholerized resist, while the others succumb or fall dangerously sick.

"Effects of the microbe in man: The injection in the region of the brachial triceps of eight drops of a very fresh virulent culture produces a painful and hot tumor that hinders the movement of the arm; the consequence of this state is a localized fever that soon disappears spontaneously; three hours after the injection the evolution of this phlegmasy begins, continues during about twenty-four hours, after which all uneasiness disappears almost completely without any phlegmon or eschar being observed.

"If five cubic centimetres are injected in each arm, the local symptoms are more marked and general symptoms appear. By observing the most salient features in each individual, we can form a general picture, the resemblance of which to true cholera is beyond dispute. . . .

"If six or eight days after the injection of five cubic centimetres the same dose with the same degree of virulence be reinjected into the same individual, the general symptoms disappear and the local symptoms are much less marked.

"From these facts, well-defined and easy to reproduce, we are justified in inferring: 1st. The possibility of cholerization in man as in guinea-pigs by means of hypodermic injections. 2d. That the prophylaxis of cholerization is obtained either by using virulent injections or with graduated doses." (FERRAN, *On the pathogenic and prophylactic action of the comma bacillus. Academy of Sciences*, 13th April, 1885.)

By comparing this note of M. Ferran with that of 18th of January, 1886, which will be found further on, we can understand why vaccinated persons have experienced morbid symptoms in the first period of choleric vaccination whereas in the last they felt none whatever.

At the time of writing the first note, M. Ferran vaccinated with strong virus, that is to say, with the living microbe.

Later on, he only vaccinated with the leucomaines of the comma bacillus. (*Note of the* AUTHOR.)

PART SECOND

DEMONSTRATION OF THE THEORY.

PART SECOND.

DEMONSTRATION OF THE THEORY.

CHAPTER I.

THE VACCINE OF FOWL-CHOLERA.

Vaccination with the attenuated virus of fowl-cholera according to the method of M. Pasteur has been the subject of several notes communicated to the Academy of Sciences at different times. In order to make their reading easier, I here transcribe as a summary of these notes the exposition of this method contained in a˙ work that has had a great success, and the exactness of which, I believe, cannot be doubted.*

"Truly, among the scourges that afflict humanity, there are none greater than the virulent distempers. Measles, scarlatina, diphtheria, small-pox, syphilis, anthrax, yellow-fever, typhoid fever, Eastern plague form a terrible enumeration, not to mention farcinus, leprosy, and rabies ! The history of these disorders presents some extraordinary circumstances. The strangest, without doubt, is that which has always been observed among a great number of them, non-recurrence. As a general rule, and notwithstanding some rare exceptions, man suffers but once from measles,

* *Histoire d'un savant par un ignorant.*

scarlatina, the plague, or yellow-fever. What explanation, even hypothetical, can be given of such a fact ? There is yet something still more surprising. How can vaccination, which is itself a virulent disease, though mild, preserve from a more serious disorder, the small-pox ? Was there ever an observation more mysterious in its causes and its origins, an observation unique in the history of medicine, and which during a whole century has baffled all comparison ?

" 'But,' reasoned M. Pasteur, having pondered for a long time on the discovery of Jenner, 'if none of the virulent diseases return, why should there not be found for each, some malady, of either a different or similar nature, which, acting on them like vaccination on small-pox, would have a preservative virtue ? ' A chance—one of those chances that present themselves to those who leave nothing undone to bring them about—allowed M. Pasteur to accomplish this progress and to make the discovery which has been justly considered one of the greatest of the century.

" Passing the microbes of fowl-cholera from one culture to another in an artificial medium, and repeating this a sufficient num. ber of times to make it impossible to imagine that the least trace of a droplet of the virulent matter which served as a starting point could be found in the last fluid, by which the virulence of the culture could be explained, M. Pasteur proved in the most absolute manner that the infectious microbes are the sole cause of the diseases that correspond to them. It is not only ten or twenty cultivations of fowl-cholera that can thus be made, but a hundred and even a thousand, and at the thousandth the virulence is neither extinguished nor even sensibly weakened. But—and this is well worthy of our attention—the virulence with successive cultures is not preserved, *unless there be no interval between one and another.* It is necessary, for instance, to plant the second culture twenty-four hours after the first ; the third, twenty-four hours after the second; the hundredth, twenty-four hours after the ninety-ninth.

If between one culture and another *several days, several weeks, and, above all, several months* are allowed to pass, a great change is observed in the virulence. The change, which generally varies according to the interval, is marked by a decrease in the energy of the virulency.

"If the broods of fowl-cholera made at very short intervals have a degree of virulence such that ten, twenty inoculated fowls perish within twenty-four or forty-eight hours, a culture that has stood three months in its breeding flask, stoppered with a wad of cotton wool in order to allow only the access of pure air, may, if inoculated on twenty fowls, make them all more or less sick, but *will not cause the death of a single one*. They will all recover after a few days of fever, sadness, and lack of appetite. But if this phenomenon be indeed extraordinary, the following is likewise so in another manner. If after the cure of these twenty fowls they be reinoculated with a very virulent virus, that for instance before mentioned as being able to kill twenty fowls in twenty-four or forty-eight hours, these fowls may perhaps become somewhat sick but will not die. The conclusion to be derived from these facts is clear. The disease can protect against itself. It has distinctly one of the characteristics of virulent diseases, that of non-recurrence.

"Curious as it may be, this character is, however, not a thing unknown to pathology. Small-pox was artificially created to preserve against the natural disease; anthrax is still produced in sheep to prevent the consequences of the same distemper; to preserve horned cattle against peripneumonia, they are inoculated with the virus of peripneumonia itself. Fowl-cholera offers an immunity of the same order. This constitutes the acquisition to science of a new fact, but there is nothing novel in the principle.

"The great novelty which is a consequence of the facts above related, and which gives them a separate place in our knowledge of virulent maladies, is that they refer to a disease the virulent agent of which is a microscopical parasite, a living being capable

of being cultivated outside the economy; and that the attenuation
of its virulency lies within the power of the experimenter, who
creates it, diminishes it, and does with· it whatever he chooses.
And all these variable virulences are obtained from the maximum
virulence, merely by a process in the laboratory.

"Similar in its action to vaccination in regard to small-pox, this
weakened microbe, which does not cause death, acts towards the
fatal microbe as a true vaccine or preservative. In fine, it brings
on a disease that may be terminated mild, since it does not occasion
death, and may preserve from the disease in its fatal form.

"But in order for this microbe to be a real vaccine such as that
of cow-pox, would it not be necessary, so to speak, that it be fixed
in its own variety, so as not to be obliged to have recourse to the
original preparation? When Jenner had fully shown that inoculated cow-pox was a protection against small-pox, he feared for
some time that to obtain the vaccine he would always have to have
recourse to the cow-pox of the cow. His real discovery consisted
in having proved that it was not necessary to have the virus direct
from the cow, the inoculation from arm to arm being sufficient.
M. Pasteur made his microbe pass from culture to culture. What
would it become? Would its virulence recover its activity or remain in its mild form?

"The virulence remained unchanged in the attenuated condition
already acquired. It was therefore a true vaccine. When this
discovery was made known, several veterinary surgeons and far-
mers applied to M. Pasteur in request of a preservative against the
distemper so fatal in poultry-yards. Trials were made with the
best possible results. To preserve this 'vaccine' it is kept from
the contact of the air in tubes with the extremities closed with the
blow-pipe.

"Before the moment in which the attenuation is reached, in the
interval placed at will between two successive cultures of microbes
that causes the attenuation and produces the 'vaccine,' what has

been going on? What is the secret of this influence? The intervening agent is in reality no other than the oxygen of the air, as we will now prove.

"If the culture be made in a tube containing very little air and the ends closed at the blow-pipe, the microbe during its growth soon absorbs all the free oxygen in the tube and that dissolved in the liquid. Thus completely preserved from the contact of oxygen, the microbe during whole months and sometimes for years will not be sensibly attenuated.

"The oxygen of the air appears therefore as the cause of the modification in the virulence of the microbe.

"But what explanation is to be given of the non-influence of the oxygen of the air on successive cultures when practised every twenty-four hours? There is only one possible in the opinion of M. Pasteur: to wit, that in this case the oxygen of the air is only employed for the life of the microbe. A cultivation lasts several days. At the end of twenty-four hours, it is not yet finished.. The air that comes in contact with the microbe is used therefore wholly for its nourishment and propagation. After that, when the cultivation is prolonged for a certain time, the air acts only as a modifier, and a moment arrives in which the attenuation is so great that the virulence disappears entirely.

"Then may be observed the extraordinary fact of the absence of virulency before the death of the microbe. The cultures offer the spectacle of a microbe that may be cultivated indefinitely, and yet be incapable of thriving in the bodies of fowls and consequently deprived of virulence." *

The microbe is a living being. In the growth of every animal or vegetable there are two totally distinct things, the germ and the complete being.

*Histoire d'un savant par un ignorant (Le vaccin du choléra des poules, page 287).

The phenomena are not the same for one as for the other. The vegetable or animal once brought to life cannot interrupt it, and must continue its functions till it dies. The length of this life is always limited.

Whereas the germ may in some cases remain for a considerable time unperceived in the state of germ, it may even perish without having lived; that is to say, it may lose its power to pass from latent to real life.

M. Pasteur says that the microbes he inoculates are attenuated, and that this attenuation is due to the action of oxygen.

To begin with, we must know what is attenuation. No explanation is given of it. It is simply said that the attenuated microbe no longer kills, and that, its properties having changed, its action becomes therapeutic.

Has the microbe wholly and entirely changed its species? Is the phenomenon, for instance, the same as if a pear-tree were changed into a cherry-tree?

This is not probable. Since the oxygen, according to M, Pasteur, is necessary to the birth and growth of the microbe we must infer that it is not only useful, but absolutely necessary to its life; for such is the case in the organisms that are best known to us.

In my opinion, the oxygen acts on the microbe in a manner much more simple and perfectly well known.

M. Pasteur introduces the microbe in broth, and allows the passage of air through a cotton stopper.

Here, the life of the microbe takes place in all its phases, both as a germ and as a living being.

Consequently in these conditions when a microbe is taken from one culture and placed in another, having again every favorable condition, it must germinate, thrive, and live, just the same as in the first culture, and so on in all the other cultures that may be innumerable.*

In these conditions of perfect life the microbes should kill the individual if they were introduced in a medium favorable to their growth, as is the case with natural contact.

Let us now see how M. Pasteur obtains attenuated virus. He leaves one of his cultivations in the broth where the microbes are bred for several weeks, and sometimes as long as three months, and when at this period the fowls are inoculated, they no longer die; they are vaccinated.

The explanation is the following:

M. Pasteur, on leaving in the same broth a cultivation of microbes, limits the elements necessary to their life, allowing but one element to be renewed, *the air which provides them with oxygen.*

What must happen then? The microbes will live until they have completely abstracted the alimentary substances that they can find in the broth, and they will die as soon as these substances are completely exhausted.†

These microbes would perish in the same manner as men shut up in an apartment; they would all become sick, and, if not at the same time, one after the other would die; not one would survive.

* Koch succeeded in cultivating during two years the bacilli of tuberculosis, and in making them pass through nearly one hundred generations without perceiving the least attenuation in their effects. *Investigations on the microbe of Asiatic cholera,* by Dr. Van Ermengen.)

† In any case the duration of life of generations proceeding from the same stock seems to be limited, the race appears to be exhausted at the end of a certain length of time, especially if the medium be not constantly renewed. (Dr. E. Van Ermengen.)

If the microbe be dead, the action of immunity cannot be attributed to it, and as the only things contained in the broth that were not there before the introduction of the microbes are the products, or in other words, the leucomaines, it must be to these products that the curative action spoken of by M. Pasteur to the Academy is to be attributed.*

The greater lapse of time between each planting of germs implies a longer period of cultivation in the same broth and consequently a less amount of nourishment for a given quantity of microbes.

If a cultivation be made in a hundred cubic centimetres of broth and the broth changed at the end of twenty-four hours, the culture of micro-organisms will have had one hundred centimetres per day.

If this cultivation be left one hundred days in the same broth, it will only have one cubic centimetre per day or one one-hundredth of the amount in the former case.

What effect has a diminution of nourishment on all living beings?

It cannot but diminish life; that is to say, must become a cause of death. This is the only phenomenon that can be produced in M. Pasteur's cultivations.

This he himself confesses when he says: "The most attenuated virus is that nearly dead."

What must necessarily happen in these cultivations that are a long time without being renewed is that in the beginning the micro-organisms perform their functions with all the activity that their powers allow, but at the end of a certain length of time, the nourishment becoming more and

* See further on, Chapter IV., *Reappearance of Virulence.*

more scarce, their life is laborious and weakened, and death will inevitably follow.*

How can we explain now what happens in the tube that M. Pasteur closes hermetically after filling it with broth and a cultivation of microbes?

The only difference between this cultivation and the former is that this one is closed, that is to say, the presence of air therein is excluded. In this cultivation there must be two distinct things: the *plant* and the *germ*. The plant, if the air is not necessary to its life, will live till all the substances in the broth that it needs are completely exhausted. If the air is necessary to it, it will die as soon as shut up.

In either case, after a longer or shorter lapse of time, it will undoubtedly perish.

But the case is entirely different as regards the germ.

If the germ require either air or oxygen to germinate, and it be deprived of one or the other, it will remain in the state of germ one or two years until the moment when it comes in contact with this vivifying element that was lacking to it.

This moment arrived, the germ will become a microbe, life will begin anew, and the cultivation made at this period will necessarily be mortal, as there will then be living microbes.

The same thing happens when wine is enclosed hermetically. This wine contains germs that remain in the state of such till the moment arrives of their coming into con-

---

* The death of the parasite is moreover an habitual and *constant* circumstance, whenever a sufficient time has elapsed between one cultivation and another. (PASTEUR, *Comptes rendus of the Academy of Sciences*, 26th October, 1880.)

tact with the oxygen of the air, as proved by Gay Lussac; and at this very moment they are transformed into myco· dermæ and produce the different fermentations distinctive of each mycoderma; the same phenomenon therefore occurs with the microbes and germs shut up in M. Pasteur's tube; they have the power to preserve their virulency.

CHAPTER II.

VACCINATION OF ANTHRAX.

"IN recent communications," says M. Pasteur,* "I have made known the first case of the attenuation of a virus by the sole means of experimentation. Composed of a special microbe of exceeding minuteness, this virus can be multiplied by artificial cultivation, outside the bodies of animals. These cultivations, left to themselves, all possibility of their contents being contaminated avoided, undergo in time modifications more or less complete in their virulence. Here it is the oxygen of the air that is the principal cause of these attenuations, that is to say, in the decrease of the facility of multiplication of the microbe; because it is evident that the virulence in its divers activities must depend on the power the parasite has of thriving within the economy.

"It is unnecessary to insist on the interest of these results and the inferences to be derived from them. To seek to diminish the virulence by rational means, is to found on experimentation the hope to prepare with active virus of easy cultivation in the body of man or of animals, a preservative virus or vaccine, with a limited capacity of thriving, but still capable of preventing the fatal effects of the former. Thus, we have dedicated all our efforts to the

* Communication to the Academy of Sciences (sitting of 28th February, 1881).

investigation of the possible generalization of the action of
the oxygen of the air in the attenuation of virus.

"The virus of anthrax, being one of the best studied,
naturally was the first to draw our attention. However,
we encountered a difficulty from the outset.

"Between the microbe of fowl-cholera and the *bacillus
anthracis* there is an essential difference that prevents the
investigation in this latter being followed up exactly in the
same manner as the former. The microbe of fowl-cholera
does not appear to resolve itself during its cultivation into
a true germ. In these cultivations, all we can observe are
cellules or articles always disposed to multiply by fission,
but the particular conditions in which true germs are produced are unknown to us.*

" Yeast of beer is a striking example of these cellular
productions that reproduce indefinitely without their spores
appearing.

"There are many mucedineæ with tubular mycelia
which, in certain conditions, produce chains of cellules
more or less spherical in shape called *conidia*. These, separated from their branches, can reproduce under the form
of cellules without ever making the spores of their respective mucedineæ appear, unless a change takes place in the
conditions of culture.

"These vegetable organizations can be compared to those
plants that multiply by shoots, and the fruit and seed of

---

* "I have before remarked that the small articulations of the
microbe resolve into granulations of a very small diameter. It is
difficult to believe that these granulations are the true germs of the
articulations, as in time the microbe dies. Can they be granulations without any life of their own?"

which are not used for the reproduction of the mother-plant.

"The bacteridia of anthrax in their artificial cultivation behave very differently. *These mycelian filaments, if they may be called so, have hardly multiplied during 24 or 48 hours, when they are observed to transform, especially those that have a free contact with the air, into ovoidal corpuscles, very refringent that can gradually isolate themselves and constitute veritable germs of the small organs.*

"*Now, observation shows that these germs, so quickly formed in the cultures, do not undergo with the lapse of time any alteration caused by contact with the atmospheric air, either in their vitality or virulence.* I could present the Academy with a tube containing spores of bacillus anthracis formed four years ago, the 21st of March, 1877. Every year I make trials of germination with the small corpuscles, and every year this germination takes place with the same facility and rapidity as at first; every year the virulence of the new cultures is tested, and they manifest no signs of decrease. With these facts, how would it be possible to attenuate the virus of anthrax by means of the action of the atmospheric air?

"The knot of the difficulty lies, perhaps, in the fact of the rapid production of germs just alluded to. Under its filamentous form, and in its multiplication by fissions, is not this organism exactly similar to the microbe of fowl cholera? That a germ in the true sense of the word, that a seed should undergo no modification from contact with the air, can be easily understood; but we can understand none the less easily, that if a change does take place, it will do so in preference in a mycelian fragment. *It is thus that a shoot of a tree or bush, if left on the surface of the ground in contact with the air, will lose its vitality in a short time, while under these conditions the seed would be preserved with its faculty to reproduce the plant.* If there is any foundation for these views, we are led to think that for the bacteridia of anthrax to experiment the action of the air, it would be necessary to be able to bring under this action the mycelian growth of the small organisms *in circumstances in which it could not furnish the smallest germ-corpuscle.* The question thus stated is, as we shall show, susceptible of being solved.

" We can, in fact, prevent the spores from appearing in he artificial cultures of anthrax by various means. At a temperature of about 16° C. (60° F.), which is the lowest at which this parasite can be cultivated, it does not give off germs, at least for a very long time. The forms of the small microbe at this inferior limit of its growth are very irregular, sometimes marble-shaped, sometimes like pears, in a word, monstrous, but unprovided with spores. The same thing happens at the highest temperatures still compatible with the cultivation of the parasite, which vary according to the medium employed.

" In neutral hen-broth, the bacteridia cannot be cultivated at a temperature of 45° C. (113° F.). But their cultivation is both easy and abundant at from 42° to 43° C. (108° to 109° F.), but there is no possible formation of spores. *Consequently it is possible to maintain in contact with pure air, between 42° and 43°, a mycelian culture of bacteridia entirely deprived of germs.*

"'Then appear the following very remarkable results: *In*

*about a month's time, the culture is dead, that is to say,
replanted in fresh broth, it is completely sterile.* The day
before this impossibility of growth manifests itself, and
during all the days previous during the month the culture
has stood, its reproduction is easy. This, as regards its life
and nutrition. As to its virulence, the extraordinary fact
is observed *that the bacteridia are deprived of it from the
eighth day ahead if the temperature is maintained between
42° and 43°.* At least, its cultures are inoffensive for the
guinea-pig, the rabbit, and the sheep—three of the animal
species most liable to contract anthrax. We can thus not
only attenuate the virulence of a disease, but suppress it
completely in appearance, simply by modifying its culture
in a certain manner.

" Besides, we can preserve and cultivate the terrible microbe in this inoffensive state. What happens during these
first eight days at 43° that suffice to deprive the bacteridia
of all virulence? We will recall the fact that the microbe
of fowl-cholera also perishes in its culture in contact with
the air, at the end of a much longer time it is true, but that
in the interval it undergoes successive attenuations. Are
we not authorized to think that the same thing may happen
with the microbe of anthrax? Experience has proved this
surmise to be true.

"Before its virulence becomes extinct, the bacillus of anthrax passes through several degrees of attenuation, and
besides, as also happens with the microbe of fowl-cholera,
each one of these states of attenuated virulence can be reproduced by culture. Finally, since, as we have proved
in one of our recent publications, anthrax never returns,
each grade of our attenuated microbes constitutes a ' vac-

cine' for the microbes of a higher grade; that is to say, is
a virus capable of producing a milder form of malady.
What, then, easier than to find in these successive grades
of virus, others capable of producing the splenic fever in
sheep, cows, horses without being mortal that will preserve
them against a later fatal attack of the disorder? We have
practised this operation with great success on sheep, and
we intend to do so again on a large scale in the Beauce at
the gathering time.

"M. Toussaint has already announced that sheep can be
preserved by preventive inoculations, but when this skil-
ful operator publishes the results of his experiments, on
which we have made deep studies yet unedited, we will
show the difference between the two methods, the uncertainty of the one and the certainty of the other. That which
we make known has besides the great advantage of being
based on the existence of virus-vaccines that can be cultivated at will, and that can be multiplied to the infinite in
the space of a few hours without having recourse to blood
infected with anthrax."*

By accepting my theory, the explanation becomes extremely easy. M. Pasteur has proved that the germ-corpuscle of bacillus anthracis does not come to life in contact
with the air. These corpuscles remained in the culture
broth ready to germinate the moment they were placed in
a new liquid.

---

*De l'attenuation des virus et de leur retour à la virulence, com-
munication by MESSRS. PASTEUR, CHAMBERLAND and ROUX, to
the Academy of Sciences, 28th February, 1881.

To have the microbes without the germs, it became, therefore, necessary to sterilize these latter. This is what M. Pasteur did, and from this moment the microbe remaining in the broth several days or weeks, unable to propagate, having its nourishment limited, must naturally perish, and the case became entirely similar to that of fowl-cholera.

CHAPTER III.

PROPHYLAXIS OF RABIES.

THE preservation from rabies or hydrophobia by means of vaccination, is a result that has justly procured both the admiration of the world and the highest honor to the savant who discovered it.

The circumstances accompanying this method and the observations just published* by M. Pasteur, are another confirmation of the new theory.

In a note sent to the Academy of Sciences, the 1st of August, 1886, M. Pasteur says that in 350 individuals inoculated with the rabies vaccine, not one has felt the *least uneasiness, nor was there a single phlegmon or abscess.*

In a speech at the Stanley Club in Paris, at a dinner given in his honor by the American colony, M. Pasteur made the following assertion:

" I have acquired the certainty that the virus of rabies is accompanied by a non-virulent matter which alone is sufficient to prolong the state refractory to the distemper."

It is therefore no longer the microbe that, acting on the economy, produces immunity; it is, according to M. Pasteur, whose authority in this matter is beyond dispute, a *non-virulent matter* which by *itself alone* produces this benefit.

* 1886.

This matter can be no other than the leucomaines of the microbe of rabies; the leucomaines necessarily accompany the microbe, and, as stated in our conclusions, must be harmless to man.

The method by which M. Pasteur prepares the vaccine against rabies consists in trephining a rabbit and inoculating under the dura mater the hydrophobic medulla of a mad dog from the street.

He then passes the virus from the first rabbit to a second, to a third, and so forth to the twenty-fifth, through all of which passages the virulence remains unchanged.

All the marrows of these rabbits being hydrophobic, he cuts them in strips a few inches long, and hangs them up in a dry air.

In these conditions the virulence of these medullæ disappears slowly, and finally is extinguished altogether. ·

It is by taking one of these pieces of medulla, dissolving it in broth, and inoculating it in an individual that this latter receives immunity.

This medulla, which is hydrophobic because it comes from a rabbit dead of rabies, must contain microbes, and therefore also leucomaines, as the virus having proliferated in the rabbit till it produced its death must necessarily have worked a change in the medium in which it was placed, and consequently has left there its leucomaines.

M. Pasteur takes a piece of this medulla and exposes it several days to the air, till the virulence is completely extinct.

In this case, there are no longer any living microbes, but still their leucomaines must be there.

Therefore, if a piece of this medulla produces immunity,

since there are no living microbes, it is to their leucomaines that this action should be attributed.

This is more or less the same explanation that M. Pasteur gives when he says: " *The virus of rabies is accompanied by a non-virulent matter that is sufficient alone to produce the state refractory to rabies.*"

Referring to M. Pasteur's experiments on rabies, we read in the *Revue thérapeutique medico-chirurgicale* pamphlet of 1st of May, 1886:

" All those suffering from bites of dogs can be declared cured. . . .

" On the contrary, the failures in the cases of bites from mad wolves have fixed M. Pasteur's attention in the highest degree. He has definitely given up the opinion that at one moment he seemed disposed to accept, that there was a specific difference between the hydrophobic virus of wolves and that of dogs—an opinion difficult to defend, since, as I have remarked, the ground remains the same in domesticity. M. Pasteur now adopts a much more plausible explanation. 'The wolf,' he says, 'has made deeper and more numerous bites; he is more furious, and often attacks his victim on the head and face; the absorption is more abundant and rapid. On this account, the period of incubation is shorter after the bites of wolves than after those of dogs.' Everybody will be disposed to accept such an explanation."

This new explanation furnished by M. Pasteur supports our opinion on the different degrees of virulence of the disease-producing microbes. As already mentioned in the chapter on attenuations of virus, there is no other difference between one class of microbes and another than their

greater or less vitality,* on account of the more or less nutritive medium in which they are placed, and no difference
between one broth and another than the larger or smaller
number of microbes and the greater or less quantity of
leucomaines they contain.

Microbes are not, as several writers on the subject maintain, in perpetual evolution, in a state of constant change.†

Since publishing the above in the first edition of the present work, M. Pasteur has had some fatal terminations,
though few in number, among those vaccinated against
rabies.

Those who died manifested none of the known symptoms
of rabies, still M. Pasteur qualified these cases as *rabies ·
paralytica.*

In view of these results, and after mature studies, M. Pasteur modified his method and adopted that known as the
intensive method, consisting in the employment for his

---

* Pasteur has stated that blood-bacilli which have become attenuated in virulence by exposure to 42° or 43° C. for twenty days
are capable of starting new cultures of attenuated virus. This I
question, for I find that such a culture starts new cultures of
virulent bacilli; in the same way the bacilli of a culture that is
only a " vaccine " for sheep, when it is inoculated into a guinea-
pig, kills it with anthrax, and then yields bacilli that are fatal to
sheep. (Dr. E. KLEIN, Micro-organisms and Disease, page 157.)

† The cultures are similar for each degree of virulence. If at
times small changes appear to be observed, they soon seem to be
only accidental, because they disappear or are produced inversely
in new cultures. (*Academy of Sciences*, 26th October, 1880.
Communicated by M. PASTEUR.

inoculations of a marrow more recently extracted from a
dead rabbit.

M. Pasteur's experiments would, therefore, lead us to
believe that a marrow containing a culture of the microbe,
say fifteen days old, is sometimes mortal, while a culture
of only three or four days is not so.

How is this phenomenon to be explained, allowing our
theory to be exact? It would really appear difficult and
even contradictory.

If we consider the marrow as a culture of this microbe,
the more days that elapse the more exhausted the medium
in which it lives will become, the greater will be the number
of leucomaïnes capable of acting as a cause of immunity,
and the smaller the number and vital power of the microbes;
therefore the cases of rabies should be fewer the older the
marrows employed. And yet the facts are in contradiction
to this assertion.

The studies of the learned Dr. Ferran have explained this
phenomenon in a way that agrees completely with my
theory.

The experiments made by this gentleman prove that the
fatal cases observed by M. Pasteur are due to the possible
contamination with the *bacillus fluorescens*, whose intoxicating action on rabbits resembles the symptoms of paralytic rabies.

Dr. Ferran thus expresses himself:

" If scientific logic, thousands of facts proved beyond a
possibility of doubt and the laws derived from them, show
clearly and distinctly that the paralytic rabies attributed to
the virus used for vaccination taken from rabbits does not

in reality exist, to what then can be due all those accidents that occasionally present themselves in individuals subjected to the anti-rabic inoculations?

"We have already shown with facts and potent reasons that the preparation of this vaccine, like that of Jenner, has the very serious defect of not being able to be obtained in a state of absolute purity; so, if we can now prove that one of the germs, that usually render impure the anti-rabic virus, can exert on rabbits a malefic influence capable of causing their death, accompanied with symptoms similar to those observed in the case of Jorba,* our original manner of considering this very important affair will be fully justified.

"On several occasions, in the examination we were making of germs that usually contaminate the virus of rabies, we have met with a chromogenic polymorphous bacillus which can be seen in the annexed cut magnified eight hundred and fifty times. This bacillus is aerobic, and by cultivating it in agar-agar it elaborates a fluorescent emerald-green pigment that changes in time to a bluish-green, and finally takes a dark tint of a dirty and undefined color; assuredly, every practical bacteriologist has more than a hundred times come across this very common microphyte known as *bacillus fluorescens*.

"The action of this microbe on rabbits is worthy of observation. The injection of the amount contained in one division of Pravaz's hypodermic syringe into the cellular tissue of the abdomen of a rabbit, causes a local phlegmasy

---

* Studies on Rabies and its Prophylaxis, by Dr. Jaime Ferran (Clinical report of the disease of Miguel Jorba, taken from data furnished by Dr. Gonzalez), Barcelona, 1888.

with limited infiltration and exudation; a slight and passing
fever accompanies this inflammation, followed by a cutaneous anæsthesia so extraordinary that the animal remains
indifferent to every stimulus, however strong. In vain may
we burn its snout, ears, toes, or any other part of the tegu-
ment; the sensible covering of the animal seems to be under
the influence of cocaine. This insensibility is accompanied
by a strong marked paralysis, the muscular contractility refusing to manifest itself even with the faradic currents or
with any other stimulus; when the paralysis has not
reached its highest degree, the movements of the animal are
tremulous and ataxic. The toxic action of this microbe
exerts such a marked influence on the crura of the cere-
bellum, that some rabbits have the movements known as
the "leaping ague," that characterize the injuries of that
part of the brain. All these symptoms are developed
within a period varying from one to eight days, according
to the amount of the dose of culture and the point of injection. Having inoculated a pure culture of this microbe in
the cellular tissue, the venous plexus, and under the me-
ninges, it was in this latter case that with an equal dose the
action was the most rapid and energetic.

Microscopic examination reveals the presence of the
chromogenic bacillus in the vicinity of the point of inoculation, but not in the blood, nor in the brain of operated
animals. This, however, is due to their scarcity, for, if
notwithstanding our failure to discover them there, a drop
of blood from the heart, or a particle of brain be sown in
agar-agar, the microbe is reproduced, thus proving that it
is diffused in a larger or smaller quantity in these tissues.

"These are the facts relating to the action of this particular micro-organism, and observe, that we, as yet, say nothing of the other microbes that may accidentally contaminate the vaccine of the virus of rabies prepared by the classic method. This consideration alone is sufficient, even should no importance be considered due to the present study, for serious and well-judging men to suspend till later on any opinion relative to the so-called *rabies paralytica* of the inoculated. As for us, we be believe that Jorba suffered from the effects of the chromogenic microbe we have been mentioning. Fortunately, this microphyte is not so fatal to man as to rabbits, which we can assert, as on examining the register of inoculated individuals we find that only three other persons treated with our primary method felt, though in a slight and very transient manner, something resembling that suffered by the professor from Masquefa. The correctness of our views is the more firmly established if we take into account that, in the cases of pretended *rabies paralytica*, no experiments have been made to prove it by inoculating on dogs and rabbits the nervous bulbs of persons having succumbed from this cause; so, therefore, it is impossible to attribute to rabies the phenomena observed, since experimental facts are wanting, and a new microphyte presents itself that, on being introduced into the system with the anti-rabic injection, produces symptoms of excitement, hyperæsthesia, paralysis and anæsthesia, and is besides capable of causing the death of animals thus affected." *

* *Studies on rabies and its prophylaxis*, by DR. JAIME FERRAN, director of the Barcelona Microbiological Laboratory (clinical report of the disease of Miguel Jorba taken from data furnished by Dr. Gonzalez, his visiting physician), Barcelona, 1888.

Mr. Helman, director of the anti-rabic laboratory established in St. Petersburg, declares, in a note addressed to M. Pasteur, that it has been impossible in any single case to obtain the *rabies furiosa* in a rabbit by inoculations from those affected with *rabies paralytica.* This fact, the importance of which will not escape the attention of any one, would appear to be a still further confirmation of the experiments made by M. Ferran. (See *Letter of M. Pasteur on rabies.* Annales de l'Institut Pasteur, 25th January, 1887.)

CHAPTER IV.

REAPPEARANCE OF VIRULENCE.

We will first quote the words of M. Pasteur on a problem of great interest, viz., the possible reappearance of virulence in virus that has been attenuated, or even in that in which it has become extinct:

" We have just seen how to obtain bacteridia of anthrax deprived of virulence for guinea-pigs, rabbits and sheep. Can their energy be returned to them as regards these animal species? We have likewise made a preparation of microbes of fowl-cholera completely deprived of any virulent action on fowls. How may we make it possible for them to be developed anew in these animals?

" The secret of these reappearances of virulence, as far as we yet know, lies entirely in successive cultures in the bodies of certain animals.

" The attenuated bacteridia, harmless to guinea-pigs, are not so at a certain age of these animals, though the period from their birth in which virulence can manifest itself is exceedingly short. A guinea-pig several years old, one year, six months, a few weeks, eight, seven, six days old, or even less, is in no danger of death, or even of becoming ill, if inoculated with the weakened bacteridia before mentioned, which, however—strange as it may seem—are fatal to a guinea-pig one day old.

"In all our experiments we have found no exception to
this rule. If the blood of one of these guinea-pigs one day
old be inoculated to a second, and that of this to a third,
and so on, the virulence of the bacteridia is progressively
strengthened; or in other words, they gradually acquire
the possibility of developing in the economy. Consequently, it will soon be possible to produce a condition of
virulence fatal to guinea-pigs three and four days old, then
to those of a week, a month, several years, and finally
even to sheep. The bacteridia will have recovered their
original virulence. Although we have not yet had the
occasion to make the experiment, we do not hesitate to
assert that they would in the end kill even cows and horses.
This state of virulence once attained persists indefinitely if
nothing is done to attenuate it anew.

" As regards the microbe of fowl-cholera, when it has become harmless to fowls, its virulence can be made to
reappear by inoculating very small birds, such as finches,
canaries, sparrows, etc., all which species it kills immediately. Then, by successive passages through the bodies of
these birds it is made to acquire slowly a virulence capable
of being manifest in grown fowls. Need I add that during
the process of endowing these micro-organisms with renewed virulence, vaccines may be prepared with any degree
of virulence for the bacteridia, and that the same thing
happens with the microbe of cholera. This question of the
renewal of virulence is of the highest interest for the etiology
of contagious remedies.

"I finished my communication of the 26th of October
last by remarking that the attenuation of virus by the in-

fluence of air must be one of the factors in the extinction of great epidemics.

"The foregoing facts will in turn explain the so-called 'spontaneous' appearance of these scourges.

"An epidemic that has become extinct by the debilitation of its virus may break out afresh if, by certain influences, the virus acquires new vigor. The accounts I have read of the spontaneous appearances of the plague appear to me to offer examples of this mode of acting; for instance, that of Bengazhi in 1856-58, the appearance of which could by no means be traced to a contagious origin.

"The plague is a virulent disorder peculiar to certain countries. In all these countries its attenuated virus must exist ready to resume its active nature when conditions of climate, famine and misery again present themselves. There are other virulent maladies that appear spontaneously in all countries. Such, for instance, is typhus or camp fever. The germs of the microbes that produce these diseases are without doubt scattered all around. Man carries them on him or in his intestinal tube without any harmful effect, but they may become dangerous when, through accumulation and successive development, on the surface of sores and ulcers in weakened bodies or otherwise, they acquire progressively fresh virulence.

"We thus behold virulence under a new light which is by no means reassuring to humanity, unless Nature during its evolution through past ages has already encountered every occasion possible for the production of virulent or contagious diseases, which is very improbable.

"What is a microscopic organism harmless to man or to a certain determined species of animals? It is a being in-

capable of developing in our body or in that of animals;
but nothing proves that, if this microscopical being were to
enter in another of the thousand and thousand species in
creation, it could not attack it and be detrimental to it.
Its virulence, then, strengthened by successive passages in
individuals of this species may become capable of being
fatal to larger beings, man, for instance, or certain domes-
tic animals. By this method, new virulencies and conta-
gions may be created. I am very much inclined to believe
that it is thus that variola, syphilis, the plague, yellow
fever, etc., have made their appearance after being apparently extinct for ages; and that it is also by phenomena
of this nature that certain great epidemics appear from
time to time, as for instance, that of typhus just mentioned.

"The facts observed when variolation (inoculation of
small-pox) was in vogue had given rise in science to the
contrary opinion, that of the possible diminution of virulence by the successive passage of the virus through certain
subjects. Jenner held this opinion, which was not at all
improbable. Still, though we have purposely looked for
them, we have not as yet found a single instance in which
this manner of acting takes place.

"These inductions will, I hope, find new proofs in pos-
terior communications.*

"In the communication to the Academy on the 28th
February last, we announced that it was easy to obtain the
bacterium of anthrax at any degree of virulence, from that
which is mortal, that is to say, fatal a hundred times in a

_____

* *De l'atténuation des virus et de leur retour à la virulence by*
MM. PASTEUR, CHAMBERLAND and ROUX. (*Academy of Sciences*,
28th of February, 1881.)

hundred to guinea-pigs, rabbits and sheep, down to the most harmless degree, passing meanwhile through numerous intermediate states. The method for preparing this attenuated virus is extremely simple, as it is sufficient to cultivate very virulent bacteridia ·in chicken broth at a temperature 42°–43° C. (108°–109° F.), and when the culture is complete to leave it in contact with the air at this same temperature. Owing to the circumstance that in these conditions *the bacteridia do not form spores, the original virulence cannot be preserved in germs, which would inevitably happen at temperatures from 30° to 40° C. (86° to 104° F.) and under. Thus prepared, the bacteridia become more and more attenuated every day, every hour, until finally the virulence is so small that we are obliged to have recourse to guinea-pigs only one day old in order to render its action at all perceptible.*

"This extremely feeble virulence so near the point of complete extinction has naturally induced us to carry our experiments still further in order to obtain, if possible, a yet greater attenuation. We succeeded in this object, commencing with the most virulent culture that till now we have had in our possession; precisely that which I mentioned in my communication of the 28th February as proceeding from the germination of germ-corpuscles of four years' standing. I was able to maintain this culture for more than six weeks at a temperature of 42°–43°. The experiment commenced on the 28th of January. By the 9th of February the culture was harmless for grown-up guinea-pigs. When the preparation had stood thirty-one days, that is, on the 28th of February, a cultivation made at 35° C. (95° F.), taken from the flask still kept at 42°–43°, was still fatal to very young mice * but not to guinea-pigs, rabbits, nor sheep.

"The 12th of March—that is to say, forty-three days after the 28th of January—a new cultivation taken from the original preparation would kill *neither mice nor guinea-pigs, not even guinea-pigs born a few hours before. We were thus in possession of a culture in which it was impossible to make the virulence reappear.* If this virulence were ever to return, we may confidently assert that it would have to be by having recourse to new species of animals yet unknown as capable of inoculation, totally distinct from those which we now know as being apt to contract anthrax.

"In other words, we now possess and have a very simple means of obtaining at will from the most virulent culture of bacteridia, others entirely harmless, exactly similar to those numerous microscopical organisms that abound in our food, our alimentary canal, the dust we breathe, without their being a cause of sickness or death, and among which we frequently seek aids for our industries." †

Here we have an experiment the result of which would at first sight seem to contradict my theory; nevertheless, we do not need a long study to find that there is nothing in it contrary to my way of considering the action of microbes.

The microbe of fowl cholera, having been attenuated till

---

* Mice are more sensitive to the action of the virus of anthrax than guinea-pigs.

† *Le vaccin du charbon* (by MM. PASTEUR, CHAMBERLAND and ROUX. (*Academy of Sciences*, 21st March, 1881.)

it no longer affects hens, is still fatal to small birds, and
by making it pass through different animals, it may again
become capable of killing hens.

The inference to be derived from this fact, namely, that
the microbe of fowl cholera is not dead, is therefore contrary to the theory I have exposed.

We pay a great attention to this point. If we admit that
the microbe in the attenuated cultures of M. Pasteur is not
dead, it ought always to be capable of reproducing the disease in the individuals of a smaller species. Nevertheless,
this is not always the fact. M. Pasteur tells us that " he
has had in his possession bacteridia in which it was impossible to renovate their virulence, and which are incapable
of killing mice or guinea-pigs, even guinea-pigs a few days
old. "

We must then conclude that when the cultures of M.
Pasteur have reached a degree of attenuation so great that
they can no longer kill mice nor guinea-pigs, that is to say,
animals infinitely smaller than those from which the first
virus was derived, they hold no living microbe, and only
contain its leucomaines; and that the degree of attenuation
of M. Pasteur's cultures depends upon the quantity of living microbes remaining in the broth.

Very attenuated broths, having very few microbes, produce in an individual sickness but not death, their number
not being sufficient to kill the subject that receives, together with the microbes, the leucomaines that are to destroy them.

The broth in which M. Pasteur prepares his culture must
therefore contain these two factors:

The microbes that are the cause of the disease, and their leucomaines that are the cause of immunity.

. The broth that only contains living microbes has the maximum of virulence, and the broth in which all the microbes are dead, and which contains the maximum quantity of leucomaines, will also have the maximum of power to give immunity.

CHAPTER V.

INHERITED IMMUNITY.

In our studies on preventive vaccinations against fowl cholera and anthrax, we have seen that the prophylactic action of the cultures of M. Pasteur must be attributed to the leucomaines contained in the culture broth.

But as these broths contain microbes either living or dead, all may not be disposed to attribute solely to the leucomaines the therapeutic action.

In support of my opinion that immunity is exclusively due to leucomaines, I have quoted the interpretation that . M. Pasteur has just given of the vaccination he practises for the cure of rabies. I have also mentioned the opinion of M. Ferran, who says that as in his broth the microbe is dead, he must attribute solely to a substance *eliminated* by the microbe the preventive action he was in search of, and which we believe to have found.

I am now going to present an experimental fact due to the investigations so intelligently carried out by M. Ch. Davaine and M. Chauveau, in which we will find a subject perfectly vaccinated and in which it is evident that a microbe has never existed.

"It is particularly on subsequent inoculations of the same nature that previous inoculations exercise an inhibitory influence. By inoculations of the same nature are meant those that are made by the same process, with the same quantity of the same infectious matter. This action, how ever, may be still more extensive. Thus, for instance, inoculation by cutaneous prickings, repeated several times, is often sufficient to neutralize, either completely or almost so, the effects of subcutaneous or even intravascular inoculations of very considerable quantities of virus.

"All these facts are certainly of great interest, but the most interesting without doubt, and which has been made manifest during my experiments on the preventive inoculations of Algerine sheep, is the one which I am now about to mention.

"In all lambs just born, the same phenomena are observed after bacteridian inoculations as among adult individuals; at times, apparent uneasiness, always an elevation of temperature in the rectum, and a swelling more or less evident in the lymphatic ganglia in the vicinity of the inoculated region. Now, none of these phenomena are observable if the mother of the young lamb has been inoculated several times during the latter months of pregnancy.

"The resistance of the young subject is then as complete as possible.

"It was on the 24th of September, 1879, that I first proved this fact in a lamb born on the 8th from a ewe that had been inoculated on the 5th and the 21st of July previous. Literally covered with inoculation prickings on different occasions, this lamb never for once presented a single trace of ganglionary tumefaction nor elevation of temperature in the rectum. The same thing happened with two other lambs, the mothers of which had been inoculated three or four weeks before lambing with considerable quantities of virus introduced by subcutaneous injections.

"From this fact, important consequences are to be derived as regards the theory of immunity either conferred or strengthened by preventive inoculations. As M. Davaine has well shown, *the small bacteridian rods do not multiply in the blood of the fœtus, even when found in prodigious quantities in that of the mother.* Moreover, the normal solid elements of the blood do not generally pass from one vascular system into the other. Active osmotic changes between the blood of the mother and that of the fœtus only occur in the plasm of the blood. We are, therefore, authorized to conclude as far as preventive inoculations of anthrax are concerned: 1st, that the direct contact of the animal system with the bacteridian elements is not absolutely necessary to make it unfit later on for their propagation; 2d, that preventive inoculations act on the humors properly so-called, rendered sterile and sterilizing, either by the abstraction of substances necessary to the bacteridian proliferation, *or rather by the addition of matters detrimental to such a proliferation.*" *

This beautiful and interesting experiment shows us that the lamb is vaccinated without there having been any bacteridia in the fœtus, even when they have existed *in prodigious quantities in the blood of the other.*

Here we have, therefore, a subject which without having

* M. CHAUVEAU, *Comptes rendus, Academy of Sciences,* 19th July, 1880.

been vaccinated cannot be affected by the malady, although belonging to a species apt to contract it.*

How is such an extraordinary phenomenon to be explained ?

What has the mother furnished to the young lamb ?

She has given it her blood and her humors.

* The following experiment again supports our theory:

"Here are, nevertheless, two facts well worthy of originating reflections on this point:

"Two heifers inoculated in November, 1880, had not become pregnant at a covering in September previous. They were again covered, and this time successfully, the one twenty days, the other three months and a half after the preventive inoculation, by a bull also inoculated at the same date and endowed with immunity. Two calves were obtained that resisted the trial as well as the five preceding ones. In this case, did the calves receive the immunity from their father or from their mother ?

"Experiments now being made, but the duration of which is long, will give us the solution of this most interesting question."

Sur la persistance des effets de l'inoculation préventive contre le charbon symptômatique et sur la transmission de l'immunité de la mère à son produit dans l'espèce bovine. (Note de MM. ARLOING, CORNEVIN, et THOMAS, Académie des Sciences, 1882, vol. XCIV., page 1396).

Very frequently, as proved by recent investigations, the microbes are transmitted through the placental circulation, and in this case the immunity of the foetus is easily explained. Sometimes, in its quality of a young being with but little resistance, it succumbs to the action of the microbe that spares the mother, and we then observe an abortion similar to that which sometimes occurs in the human species (syphilis, small-pox, etc.), as often happens in vaccinations of anthrax in pregnant cows.

But this natural transmission of the microbe does not always take place, does not even seem to be the general rule, and still, the transmission of immunity in a more or less marked degree does seem to be a general law. (Le Microbe et la Maladie, by E. DUCLAUX.)

This blood and these humors must contain a substance harmful to the proliferation of the bacteria, or else is lacking in some substance necessary to it.

This last hypothesis is not admissible, as we have several times already said; for if the blood did not contain all the substances of blood proper to its species before contracting the malady, it would no longer be the blood that the lamb required to live and thrive.

Blood in its natural state cannot contain superfluous substances, whilst, on the other hand, the same substances that are absorbed by the microbe for its nourishment are necessary to the life of the individual.

When a culture of these microbes is to be made, we must, in order to prepare it, look for substances that have a certain importance in the organism. Moreover, in the disease it is plainly to be seen that the microbe does not take from the economy secondary elements but those of essential importance, as it is the absorption of these substances that produces disease and death.

If, then, it be not the absence of any substance that produces the immunity in the lamb, it must necessarily be the presence of some substance in the blood and humors of the mother that has effected this inoculation.

This is the opinion of M. Chauveau, and it also the explanation that naturally follows from all that we have said, that this substance can be no other than the leucomaines produced by the bacteridia, and communicated to the lamb through the blood of its mother.

CHAPTER VI.

CAN leucomaines be considered as the cause of immunity in all the methods of vaccination that are known to us?

I think they can.

The principal methods of vaccination may be reduced to three:

That in which mortal virus is inoculated, that is, virus containing living microbes, into a medium unfavorable for its propagation in the animal system.

This is the system of variolization in practice before Jenner's discovery, the same that is employed in certain diseases of animals, and that which M. Ferran tells us he practised in the beginning.*

We have already said that in this system, the production of leucomaines takes place directly in the blood or the tissues of the subject we wish to endow with immunity, and that in this case, the phenomenon is exactly the same as when immunity is conferred by the disease itself.

The second method is that of attenuations obtained by means of cultures.

If the only object of these cultures were to produce leucomaines, they should only be used when the microbes no

---

* Academy of Sciences, 13th April, 1885.

longer exist, and in this case, no morbid symptoms would be observed. *

It may be said that in the manner they have been made up to the present, giving excellent results, they do produce morbid symptoms, and that it is not perfectly clear that were these symptoms not to exist the same favorable result would be attained.

To prove my theory, I must take as granted the two following suppositions, which I hope will not be disputed.

1st. On inoculating with a liquid containing an attenuated culture, if the inoculation occasions morbid symptoms, these must be attributed to the introduction into the animal organism of living microbes † in a smaller or larger number, which by their vital functions produce these localized troubles.

2d. When no morbid symptoms are observed, it is either because no living microbes have been introduced into the system, or else, because on entering it they perish before having had time to disturb it by means of their vital functions.

In vaccination by means of attenuated virus, it is generally admitted that it is necessary to strengthen the immu-

---

* I must here remark that in the conclusions which are the summary of the theory, object of the present work, as likewise in this case, I do not pretend to say that all leucomaines are harmless to the vaccinated animal ; but they are so, 1 believe, when, after recovering from the disease due to the microbes that produce these leucomaines, the individual enjoys at the same time immunity and health. (Note by the AUTHOR).

† There has nevertheless been a growth of microbes, since there has been disease, and in fact, the microbes can be found at the seat of inoculation and throughout the tissues during the course of the disease. (DUCLAUX, *Le Microbe et la maladie*.)

nity obtained from a first inoculation by two or three successive ones. *

The first inoculation is characterized by the presence of morbid symptoms, the second by symptoms that almost escape our notice or by their total absence. The third or fourth inoculation, if performed, is likewise devoid of symptoms.

Therefore, from what we have previously said, the symptoms of the first vaccination are to be attributed to the presence of living microbes; the absence of symptoms in the following vaccinations being due to the absence of living microbes, or to their death immediately on entering the animal organism, before they have had time to disturb it.

Very respectable authorities have proved that immunity is increased by second inoculations,† and as we believe to

* Finally, if we vaccinate twenty other hens with very attenuated virus, not once or twice, but three or four times, there will be no mortality whatever from inoculation of a very virulent virus, nor even disease. In this latter case, the immunity is complete, and has attained its maximum. (DUCLAUX, *Le Microbe et la Maladie*, page 163).

† This being admitted, I can assert from numerous experiments that the effects of vaccination vary with the hens; in some, one preventive inoculation with attenuated virus being sufficient to make them resist a subsequent inoculation of very virulent virus, while in others, two, or even three preventive inoculations are necessary to obtain this result; *but in every case, each preventive inoculation has an effect of its own, as it always protects in a certain degree.* In a word, vaccination can be practised in every degree, and in every case vaccination can be made complete, that is to say, the fowl can be made to resist the slightest effects of the most virulent virus. (PASTEUR, *Comptes rendus, Academy of Sciences,* 26th April, 1880.

What are the effects of the first inoculation? Of course, I do

have proved that the microbe being dead cannot be the cause of immunity, in this case, this benefit can be attributed to nothing but the leucomaines.

The actual method of inoculation is a mixed one, partaking of the two systems just exposed in our conclusions, of that in which microbes are introduced, and of that in which the leucomaines are inoculated.

The third method consists in the attenuation of the virus by its passage through living species. This method, in my opinion, is identical with the second, and all we have said of this may be applied to that now mentioned. The broths of artificial cultivation are substituted by the blood and the tissues of guinea-pigs, rabbits, etc.

The microbe inoculated into a guinea-pig must either

not count the cases, which, though possible, are extremely rare, in which the inoculation by cutaneous prickings has caused the death of animals from splenic fever. A certain number of subjects lose their liveliness and their appetite, and thus it is very easy to see at first that the inoculation has made them sick. A much larger number continue eating and ruminating as if in perfect health, and seem to have escaped completely the action of the infectious agent. But this is not at all the case, for a careful observation shows the existence of both local and general disturbances, common to all the inoculated animals, whether they show or not any sign of uneasiness. These disturbances are the increase of temperature throughout the body, and the swelling of the lymphatic ganglia that receive the afferent vessels from the inoculated region. . . .

Thus, even on the refractory Algerine sheep, the inoculation of bacilli anthracis always produces noticeable effects, swelling of the lymphatic ganglia in the vicinity of the inoculated region, increase of the general temperature, with or without signs of derangement, such as torpor and anorexia.

Let us now examine what happens when all the phenomena of the first inoculation having disappeared, a second one is made followed by several others. The consequences of these new inocula-

proliferate in the tissues of this animal or else perish.* If it does not die, if it lives in this medium composed of living tissues, of the blood and humors of the guinea-pig, it must necessarily be by extracting from these all the substances necessary to its life, and the products of this life will thus be left in this same organism. If the blood of this guinea-

tious do not resemble in any way those of the first ; the animals do not seem at all affected by this new contact with the infecting agents of the disease.

This innocuity is particularly striking in those subjects which were the most affected by the first inoculation. They not only preserve their liveliness and appetite which they lost in the first inoculation, but besides, there is no noticeable swelling of the ganglia, and the most that can be observed is a slight and very brief increase of temperature in the rectum.

The first inoculation requires a certain time to exercise its preventive action against the effects of subsequent ones. When the reinoculations are practised too soon, the consequence, as a rule, is that their effects are simply added to those of the first inoculation. On the sixth or seventh day the influence of this first inoculation is sometimes already evident; but it is principally after the fifteenth day that this influence is distinctly established.

The repetition of inoculations has always seemed to me to further insure the increase of the natural immunity. I have yet at the present moment some Algerine sheep that from the month of June, 1879, up to April, 1880, have been inoculated seven or eight times ; inoculations that are made now have absolutely no effect. (*Comptes rendus, Academy of Sciences*, Paris, 19th July, 1880. Note by M. CHAUVEAU.)

* Davaine's bacteria of septicæmia.

Dowdeswell has shown that when blood is thoroughly sterilized (*i. e.*, when the bacteria are killed), it has no longer any infective power.

But it has been shown by Gaffky and Dowdeswell that there is no increase in the virulence of the virus when it is passed through successive animals, as was maintained by Coze and Feltz (*Microorganisms and Disease*, by DR. E. KLEIN, page 93.)

pig be inoculated into another subject, the phenomena to
which this new inoculation will give rise, whether they be
immunity bestowed on the new animal or making it sick
and causing its death, must be attributed either to the presence of micr xes or to that of the leucomaines that are to
be found in t e blood of the guinea-pig. We know already
beforehand t, it the blood of this guinea-pig of itself, that
is to say, wit ut either microbes or leucomaines, will not
produce any enomenon similar to those of the inoculations we are aking of.

The case is herefore necessarily the same as that of cultivation of t microbe in a broth, because, while living in
this broth, t microbe must deposit therein its products of
elimination id the action of this broth when inoculated
on an indiv al must also be attributed to the presence of
the microb r their leucomaines; for we know that broth
in which n icrobes have been introduced and cultivated
will not gi rise to any of the symptoms we are in search
of when in ilated on subjects of any species whatever.

Microbe: e know, are extremely sensitive to the nature
of the cult -medium.

"Some them thrive very well in veal broth, while
they peris) in that made with beef.

"Still 1 re remarkable is the case of the microbe of
'rouget,' hich, according to the experiments of M. Cornevin, re ires a broth recently prepared, and dies when
placed in the same broth if too old. We must not then be
surprised to see certain attenuated microbes prefer sheep;
certain others, guinea-pigs; nor that the most virulent bacteridia which are fatal to sheep in France spare those from
lgiers which are of another race."

These are the words of M. Duclaux, and what he states is well proved.*

Microbes when coming into very favorable media will thrive and propagate extensively, and if inoculated in these conditions, will produce a very virulent ' rus. If the blood and tissues of the organism of an anim. be not very ' favorable to the microbe, it will live awhile but will die sooner, and then the only action produced ll be that of its leucomaines. According to the formula w admitted, it will be said that the virus by its passag' hrough this species has been *attenuated;* the real fact however, is rather that there will be no living microbes, (very few.

In reality, therefore, there is no essential Terence between the two methods.

* *Le Microbe et la Maladie,* page 172

CHAPTER VII.

In fowl-cholera, as likewise in anthrax, we have seen that the method of vaccination practised by M. Pasteur does not consist in attenuating the microbe in the sense in which this word is used, but only in diminishing its life, or in killing it altogether by leaving its leucomaines in the broth.

There are other systems of attenuation invented and put in practice by various scientists.

M. Duclaux recapitulates some of them that may be studied more seriously in the Reports of the Academy·of Sciences, but the essential facts of which are perfectly pointed out in the work lately published by the gentleman just mentioned.

"ACTION OF HEAT.—The series of proofs of this fact will be the study in series of the processes of attenuation which we have at present at our disposal.

"Take, for instance, heat.

"Heat, as we know, when excessive kills all microbes. Between the temperature most favorable to their cultivation and that which is mortal to them, there is a zone of attenuation well studied by M. Chauveau in his investigations of the bacteridia of anthrax. The duration of the

application of heat must be in inverse ratio to the degree of
temperature, and in direct proportion to the attenuation to
be attained.

"A few facts will show us how far this law of M. Chauveau is true.

"The bacteridia in the blood of a guinea-pig dead of
anthrax can no longer be inoculated if the blood has been
subjected to a heat of 55° to 60° C. (131°-140° F.). At 52° C.
(127° F.), from fourteen to sixteen minutes of heating are
necessary to extinguish completely the vitality in the virus.
At fourteen minutes, the virulent activity of the bacteridia
still exists, though much attenuated. It is less and less so
when the heating has lasted but twelve, ten, eight, six
minutes. At 50° C. (122° F.), twenty minutes are necessary
to kill the bacteridia, eighteen to attenuate it in a high degree, while it still retains a great virulence if only heated
for ten minutes.

"The attenuation, as was to be expected, corresponds to
the degree of debility to which the activity of proliferation
of the microbe is reduced. If comparative cultures are
made, in a conveniently prepared fluid, with unheated
blood of animals infected with anthrax, and quantities of
the same blood heated to 52° during eight, nine, ten, to
sixteen minutes respectively, the delay in the growth is
hardly perceptible in blood heated during eight, nine, and
ten minutes, as compared with the first cultivation serving
as type; in that of eleven minutes, it is already remarkable;
more and more so as we approach the cultivations of blood
heated for fifteen minutes, in which the growth is very
problematical, while in the last there is none whatever.

"ACTION OF THE SUN.—Next to the action of heat, that of the light of the sun naturally follows. It kills the microbe after a certain length of time of exposure, but before causing its destruction it attenuates it. This is the result of my experiments, confirmed by those of M. Arloing.

"CHEMICAL ACTION OF OXYGEN.—We have seen the mode of action of physical agents; we will now examine chemical actions.

"Oxygen is a physiological factor of the highest importance, and we have already examined its action under this relation. But it plays a part more exclusively chemical, a toxic part, which M. P. Bert has made clearly evident.

"All microbes need small quantities of oxygen, and suffer when too much is given to them. Those that are anaerobic only require bare traces and die in common air. If aerobic, microbes live in common air, but perish in compressed oxygen. Between the physiological and toxic limits there is a zone of attenuation studied by M. Chauveau in bacteridia of anthrax.

"ACTION OF ANTISEPTICS.—Next to oxygen, we naturally study the action of antiseptics which, when in small quantities, do not act at all or even are favorable to microbes, but are fatal to them in higher doses. MM. Chamberland and Roux have studied the action of carbolic acid, bichromate of potash, and sulphuric acid on the bacillus anthracis.

"A very moderate dose of these three antiseptics—$\frac{1}{500}$ of carbolic acid, $\frac{1}{1700}$ of bichromate—will impede the reproduction of the bacteridia which perish in a very short time. Smaller doses—$\frac{1}{600}$ of carbolic acid, $\frac{1}{2000}$ of bichromate—

allow the growth of the bacillus in filaments, but stop its
power of reproduction, just the same as the temperature of
43° practised by M. Pasteur, by preventing its giving off
spores. From this moment the same mechanism comes
into play, and a gradual attenuation is going on apace with
the weakening of the microbe till the moment of its death." *

As M. Duclaux himself recognizes, the idea which is a
consequence of all these systems is " that in a general manner the attenuation is one of the forms of the gradual debilitation of a cellule of the microbes as it approaches its
death."

It is then, according to all micrologists, in a state capable
of producing immunity by inoculation.

As with the greater number of these elements death can
be produced suddenly, there is a notable difference between
these systems and that practised by M. Pasteur in the
treatment of fowl-cholera and anthrax.

M. Pasteur places these microbes in a medium with a
limited supply of nourishment; in these conditions the
microbes will not die until after having lived during the
time necessary to exhaust all the substances they are capable of abstracting from the fluid. As this alimentation
implies the elaboration and elimination of the products of
the microbes, when these die they will necessarily have left
a considerable quantity of leucomaines in the culture-
broths of M. Pasteur.

But in the attenuations by the other systems the state of
affairs is different.

* E. DUCLAUX: *Le Microbe et la maladie*, page 168 and following.

The microbe, subjected to a temperature of 55° to 60° that it is unable to support, dies instantly * without therefore, having had time to leave behind its leucomaines, as it has not had time to live.

Consequently, the microbe sown in broth and killed by heat, in the manner above described, cannot produce any disease, nor the broth containing it confer any immunity.

If by means of a convenient temperature the microbe be left in that state described by M. Duclaux as that in which "a delay in the growth is observed which becomes later on problematic if the microbe is placed in another nutritious fluid," the microbe in this case has a life similar to that of the bacillus of fowl-cholera in one of M. Pasteur's cultures, —that, for instance, of two months' standing. In these conditions it will elaborate, though in small quantities leucomaines, and these will be the cause of immunity.

Or else these microbes which will have lost the faculty of reproduction, as we have already seen is the case when subjected to the action of antiseptics, will have life sufficient, when introduced into the system, to provide it with all the leucomaines necessary to produce immunity, without causing death, on account of their weakness and of the presence of these leucomaines.

The method of attenuation by heat invented by M. Toussaint, according to a note presented in his name by M. Chauveau, consists in heating the infected blood of a sheep dead of Chabert's disease; this blood, in which the bacteria

* In a bottle containing wine and air, when heated to a temperature of from 50° to 60°, the wine never sours; it is because by the heat the germs of the *mycoderma aceti* held in suspension by the wine and air lose all their vitality. (*Histoire d'un savant par un ignorant*, p. 91.)

of anthrax have lived, since they have caused the death of
the sheep, must necessarily have undergone a change in
these conditions.   In effect, the microbe, on taking for its
nourishment some of these substances, must have deposited
therein its leucomaines.

Therefore, when this blood is heated, it is in order to
destroy the bacterium or, at least, to render its life more
feeble and to prevent its thriving when introduced, by way
of inoculation, into another organism.

As regards the system of attenuation by compressed oxygen, the explanation must be similar.   Both M. P. Bert and
M. Chauveau tell us that with this element microbes can be
killed, and that between the physiological and toxic limits
there is a zone of attenuation.*

M. Chauveau says, in his note to the Academy, that by
means of oxygen and moderate pressure, Davaine's bacillus
becomes more virulent, while under high pressure it becomes totally inactive.†   .

As oxygen is an element of life, we can understand that
this increase of virulence can only be attributed to a greater

* M. Paul Bert, in his fine works on the employment of oxygen
at high pressures as a process of physiological investigation, recognized that compressed oxygen rapidly causes the death of all living
beings.   (Note by MM. ·PASTEUR and JOUBERT, *Academy of Sciences*, 16th July, 1877—*Le charbon et la vaccination charbonneuse
d'après les travaux recents de M. Pasteur*, by CH. CHAMBERLAND,
page 28.)

† It has in effect happened that cultures of this bacillus, in contact with air or compressed oxygen, have shown, under moderate
pressure, greater activity than in the normal state, whereas a
higher pressure has rendered them completely inactive.   (*Comptes
rendus, Acad. of Sciences*, 19th May, 1884, note by M. A. CHAU-
VEAU.

vitality of the microbe, and that its inactivity must be due to its death.*

Heat, compressed oxygen, the sun and antiseptics are all in this case causes that lead to death.†

As the object of all these elements, all these methods and systems, is to act against the vitality of the microbe, we must infer that the microbes of the different maladies inoculated by these methods, when in their normal condition, kill the individual.

That when they have undergone the action of these attenuations they have lost the conditions of their normal state; that is to say, they can no longer reproduce, or their reproduction has become difficult.

If microbes in such a state be introduced into an organism, while they live there they will change the medium in which they exist till their life becomes extinct. And as we can then conceive the possibility and the probability of the existence of leucomaines, while it is impossible to conceive that of microbes which must be dead, or otherwise

---

* I have further discovered in this series of studies another very important fact. These cultures, in which *the attenuation is so absolutely certain that they will not cause the death of a single sheep, and in which the activity is so great that they confer the most solid immunity,* possess yet another great advantage: that of preserving this activity for several months. (*On the attenuation by compressed oxygen, Academy of Sciences,* 19th May, 1884, A. CHAUVEAU.)

† From all the studies that succeeded the labors of M. Toussaint on virulent attenuation by the moderate action of physical and chemical agents destroyers of virus, it is clearly evident that these agents all possess more or less the faculty of decreasing the infectious activity of the virulent ferments, instead of destroying it completely, *if care is had not to make use of all the destructive influence* to which these ferments are exposed. (*Comptes rendus, Academy of Sciences,* 19th May, 1884. Note by M. A. CHAUVEAU.)

the individual would become sick, we must in this case attribute the immunity solely to leucomaines.

If the elements of attenuation above mentioned, sun, oxygen, etc., be applied to the blood of an individual suffering from the complaint we wish to preserve against, or on a culture-broth in which the microbe has lived, we can understand yet more easily that the destructive action of these elements, even without the knowledge of the vaccinator, has had for its object to allow the leucomaines to exert their beneficent action.

CHAPTER VIII.

THE ANTIDOTE THEORY.

In treating of the several theories by which the immunity existing after a first attack of an infectious disease is explained, Dr. Klein refutes successfully that known as the *Exhaustion Theory*, which we have already several times mentioned. He proves its falsity and its inability to explain the phenomenon of immunity from a second attack, co-existent with a state of perfect health.

After this, the author sets forth Klebs' Antidote Theory, to which he adheres as being the only one in harmony with the facts.

According to this theory, immunity, as M. Chauveau had foreseen in his experiments on Algerine sheep described in a former chapter,* is due to the presence of a new substance in the animal organism.

The antidote theory has many points of similarity with that we now sustain, and on account of this resemblance upholds our theory.

We copy from Klein's work the following passages on on this subject:

"This something then, which inhibits the growth and multiplication of the bacillus anthracis in the tissue of the pig but not in the

* See Chapter V.

mouse, must be something which, although dependent on the life of the tissue, is not identical with any of the characters constituting the life of the tissue, but must be some product of that life. To assume, then, as is done by some observers, that the living state of the cells *per se* is the inhibitory power does not cover the facts, as we have just seen. The most feasible theory seems to me to be this, that this inhibitory power is due to the *presence of a chemical substance* produced by the living tissues. It does not require a great effort to conceive, and it does not seem at all improbable, that the blood and tissues of the pig contain certain chemical substances which are not present in the mouse—substances which, like so many others, chemistry is not yet capable of demonstrating. But that there exist vast and gross differences in the chemical constitution of the blood and tissues of different species of animals there can be no reasonable doubt; it is a fact with which physiological chemistry is quite familiar.

"We arrive then, after all this, at the conclusion that, owing to the presence in the blood and tissues of particular chemical substances, present only during life, and a result of the life of the tissue, the organisms in a particular case cannot thrive and produce the disease. And further, that for each particular species of organism, there is a particular chemical substance required to exert this inhibitory power, for, as we have seen, while the anthrax-bacillus is not capable of thriving in the pig, it does well in the guinea-pig; while the bacillus of swine-plague thrives well in the pig, it does not in the guinea-pig.

"The incapability of non-pathogenic organisms to thrive in healthy living tissues would on this theory be explained by the assumption that these chemical substances present in every healthy tiliving ssue are inimical to all putrefactive organisms. . . .

"There is another theory, commonly spoken of as the *Antidote Theory* (Klebs). According to this, the organisms growing and

multiplying in the body during the first attack produce, directly or
indirectly, some substance which acts as a sort of poison against
a second immigration of the same organism. I am inclined to
think that this theory is in harmony with the facts. There is
nothing known from the observations before us which would
negative the possibility of the correctness of this theory ; nay, I
would almost say all our knowledge of the life of micro-organisms
points to the conclusion that the different species are associated
with different kinds of chemical processes, and that as a result of
the activity we find different chemical substances produced.

"The different fermentations connected with the different species
of fungi afford striking illustrations of this view. According to
this theory, we can well understand that just as in the case of an
animal, say a pig, unsusceptible to anthrax—the unsusceptibility
being due to the presence in the blood and tissues of a particular
chemical inimical to the growth of the bacillus anthracis—so also
in the case of a sheep or ox that has once passed through anthrax
—there is now present in the blood and tissues a chemical substance
inimical to the growth and multiplication of the bacillus anthracis
whereby these animals become possessed of immunity against a
second attack of anthrax.

"Whether this chemical substance has been elaborated directly
by the bacilli, or whether it is a result of the chemical processes induced in the body by the bacilli during the first illness, matters
not at all; it is only necessary to assume that the blood and tissues
of the living animal contain this chemical substance.

"Some observers (Grawitz, etc.) are not satisfied with this theory,
but assume that owing to the first attack the cells of the tissues so
change their nature that they become capable of resisting the immigration of a new generation of the same organism. There is absolutely nothing that I know of in favor of such a theory ; it is impossible to imagine that the cells of the connective tissues, of the
blood and of other organs, owing to a past attack of scarlatina, be-

come possessed of new functions or of some new power, as for instance, a greater power of oxidizing or the like. Connective-tissue cells, blood-corpuscles, liver-cells and other tissues are, so far as we know, possessed of precisely the same characters and functions after an attack of scarlatina as before.

"On the whole, then, we may, it seems, take it as probable, that, owing to the presence in the normal blood and tissues in a living animal of a chemical substance inimical to the growth of a particular micro-organism, this animal is unsusceptible to the disease dependent on the growth and multiplication of this micro-organism; and further, that in those infections maladies in which one attack gives immunity against a second attack of the same kind, one attack produces a chemical substance in the blood and tissues which acts inimically to a new immigration of the same organism; hence the animal becomes insusceptible to a new attack, or is "protected." This is not the case with all infectious maladies, for, as is well known, in a good many instances a single attack does not protect against a second ; and, as is also well known, a first attack may protect but only for a limited period, or for a period greatly differing in different individuals. All this would be explained by our theory in the same way as it is explained by the other theories viz., when one attack does not protect, no inhibitory chemical substance has been produced ; which in those diseases in which one attack does protect only for a limited period, the necessary inhibitory substance has only lasted for a limited period, and so on." *

Klein therefore thinks that the natural state of resistance which certain animal species manifest against an infectious disease, is the effect of the presence of certain substances produced by the living tissues of these individuals.

He likewise believes that in animals having had an in-

* *Micro-organisms and Disease*, by DR. E. KLEIN, pp. 247–256.

fectious disease, the microbe that produced it has also produced, directly or indirectly, a substance that inhibits the proliferation of a similar microbe the second time ; and if after the disease there is no immunity from a second attack, he says this substance has not been formed.

As in our belief—the conviction of which we hope to have conveyed to the reader—the substance causing immunity is the leucomaine of the microbe that causes the disease, we cannot admit the fact of the non-elaboration of this substance, as it is a necessary consequence of the life of the microbe. What we can, should, and do admit, is that this substance will sooner or later disappear. If it disappear as soon as formed, the individual having suffered from the disease will enjoy no immunity from a second attack. If this substance disappear at the end of a month or a year, the immunity will also have lasted a month, a year, etc.

The causes of the cessation of immunity may be numerous; it may disappear through the destruction of the substance that produces it, this destruction being due to the chemical action of another substance that may be elaborated by living tissues or introduced through the alimentary canal.*

---

* M. Raulin has cultivated *aspergillus niger* in a fluid composed of several substances in known quantities. On studying the action that each one of these substances exerts on the growth of the plant, he says: "Iron seems to be only useful on account of its destroying or annihilating a poison secreted by the plant as this goes on forming. Were this poison to accumulate in the fluid, it would finally kill it. This poison is one of those excretions produced by all living beings, and which they must rid themselves of at any price. The iron renders this service to the aspergillus." (*Le Microbe et la Maladie*, by E. DUCLAUX, page 69.)

This immunity may also disappear sooner or later, either on account of the special nature of the leucomaine itself, or on account of the locality in which it was deposited by the microbe.

If we imagine it placed in a tissue destined to eliminate the products of the secretion of the animal, it is probable that the leucomaine will also be promptly eliminated.

We can understand that some leucomaines rapidly disappear from the organism owing to their own nature, by observing the phenomenon of alcoholic fermentation. (We have already seen in what this fermentation consists.) The mycoderma saccharomyces elaborates in large quantities alcohol and carbonic acid. These two substances are therefore its leucomaines.

Now, then, the alcohol, being liquid, remains behind in the place in which it has been produced, while the gaseous carbonic acid disappears, escaping thus from the presence of its generator and the fluid in which it was elaborated.

In the case of species of animals refractory to a disease, Klein believes that the immunity is likewise owing to a substance produced by their tissues.

We will not in this case venture to assert such a conclusion; we believe rather that it would be more prudent to admit that the immunity may be owing as well to the absence of a certain substance as to the presence of this same substance.

Let us suppose a liquid composed of twelve substances all necessary in order to make a cultivation of the microbe of fowl-cholera, for instance.

If we prepare a fluid containing only eleven of these substances, the microbe will not propagate. If to the fluid containing the twelve substances, we add another that will be detrimental (such as nitrate of silver for aspergillus niger)* the microbe will not thrive in this fluid either.

In those species in which microbes have never been able to propagate, the cause of the immunity should, in our opinion, be due as much to the presence as to the absence of some given matter.

But in the species in which microbes do thrive, we are forced to admit that when immunity is acquired, it is due to the addition of some substance to those naturally present in the individuals of this species.

* See Chapter III., Part 3d. Experiment of M. Raulin.

CHAPTER IX.

WINES AND BEERS.

Yeast, which produces alcoholic fermentation, is in real
ity a living being, with all the complexity belonging to
such. This yeast contains, in small quantities, nitrogenous
matters, the elements of which are derived in part from the
sugar, part from the sal ammoniac; and principally from
the hydro-carbonates, all the elements of which are taken
from the sugar. It is, therefore, in fact, from sugar that it
has derived almost all the materials of its tissues, and what
has been abstracted for this object naturally cannot undergo alcoholic fermentation.

A small portion of this sugar, that we may estimate at
about 1% of the total weight, produces neither alcohol nor
carbonic acid: it produces yeast.

The results of Lavoisier cannot, therefore, be exact, and
M. Pasteur has even shown that they are much less so than
would be imagined. Carbonic acid and alcohol are not, in
effect, as was believed till now, the *only* products of alcoholic fermentation. A little more than 3% of the sugar is
turned into glycerin, about 1% into succinic acid.

Altogether, about 5% of the sugar does not form a part of
the equation of Lavoisier, of this splitting up into equal
parts of alcohol and carbonic acid which the remaining 95%
of the sugar undergoes, when the fermentation takes place
in ordinary conditions.

Now, indeed, this phenomenon has no longer for us the simple aspect that we first found in it, and which we naturally attributed to the simplicity of its cause.

It can no longer be a question of a simple chemical displacement of the molecules of the sugar. Out of the elements of this molecule we behold the formation of yeast, in its turn composed of nitrogenous matter, cellulose, fatty matter.

At the same time, the sugar undergoes a great many different transformations, becoming carbonic acid, alcohol, glycerine, succinic acid, and giving rise in smaller proportions to other bodies that I could mention, and even some yet unknown, *i. e.*, that science has not yet isolated, as there is no chemistry more difficult than that of living beings. In place of the chemical problem that Lavoisier thought to have solved, we see arise a physiological problem much more complex, more delicate, but also grander. and more fertile in consequences.

Fermentation is, therefore, the consequence of the nutrition and life of a micro-organism, of the *saccharomyces vini*, and the alcoholization of the must of grapes is performed by means of an aerobic being, the principal products of elimination of which are alcohol and carbonic acid.*

* But in every case these ptomaines are observed to be *the products of putrid fermentation which is always produced in dead bodies by special microbes.* The ptomaines are in this case the result of the work of the microbes of putrefaction, and are *elaborated by them in exactly the same way as the alcohol and carbonic acid of alcoholic fermentation are elaborated by yeast,* at the expense of the sugar in the fluid in which they live and multiply. (*Les Microbes, les ferments et les moisissures,* by DR. E. L. TROUESSART, page 230.)

The expression *ptomaine* is here made use of by Trouessart in a

M. Alph. Rommier has made some very interesting experiments in order to prove that the activity of the fermentation depends in part on the quantity of ferment employed.*

Let us now endeavor to find out by what means this fermentation may be arrested.

sense similar to that of leucomaine, which we have adopted. (Note by the AUTHOR.)

* "From what we are informed, for several years back a new method of vinification has been tried in Germany, in which the must of grapes, being previously sterilized, is planted with a selected yeast.

"This new style of wine-making is nothing more than the application to wine of the method of Pasteur for the manufacture of beer. It must certainly give good results, as it prevents the simultaneous production of the secondary fermentations; but the previous sterilization of the must appears to us a delicate operation and very difficult to carry out in the manufacture of wine on a large scale. - Reflecting on the application of the process, we have reasoned whether the sterilization of the must was in reality necessary for its success, and whether, by sowing a cultivated wine yeast, the commencement of the fermentation would not be hastened, thus sufficiently checking the formation of secondary fermentations.

"It has, in effect, been recognized that fermentations do not take place simultaneously in the same fluid with equal energy; the moment soon arrives in which the most intense predominates over all the others, and finally checks them altogether. It was on this principle that M. Pasteur founded his method of ferment-culture. The seeds of ferment existing in the pellicle of the grape require a certain length of time, according to the degree of heat, in order to germinate and produce wine-yeast. Meanwhile, the false yeasts and moulds are formed which, during their growth, give rise to secondary reactions that affect the quality of the wine. But if at the same moment that the grape is crushed an active wine-yeast were introduced into the must—a yeast purified by cultivation—the vinous fermentation would immediately set in, and with its

According to our theory, a very simple means exists, without depriving the liquid of any of the elements necessary to the fermentation.

If the fermentation be due to the vital functions of a microbe, it is the life of this microbe that must be put an end to, and to attain this, according to what we have already several times said, it must be put in contact with its own leucomaines—alcohol for instance.

This is exactly what is done in practice.

action would paralyze the germination and growth of the other germs.

"Acting on this idea, we established last autumn a series of fermentations, the results of three of which are reported below.

"Each one was composed of four kilogrammes of crushed chasselas (a species of grape), placed in a flask closed with a cork, with a glass tube run through it so arranged as to collect the gases.

"Flask No. 1, which served as a point of comparison, contained nothing but the grapes.

"In flask No. 2, to the four kilogrammes of grapes were added sixty centigrammes of must containing yeast of wine that had reached its second culture; while in flask No. 3, the same quantity was used of yeast that had been kept a year.

"The fermentations lasted from the 7th to the 14th of September, and were made at the ordinary temperature ranging from 15° to 22° C. (59° to 74° F.).

"The cap in flask No. 1 did not commence to form until after forty-eight hours, from which time till the 14th of September the fermentation was very slow, giving off from two to three bubbles of carbonic acid per minute. On the 14th of September, seeing that this experiment was not yet finished, while the others were, the flask was placed in a stove heated to 35° C. (95° F.), where it finished in three days, giving forth at this temperature one hundred and six bubbles of carbonic gas per minute. The experiments in flasks Nos. 2 and 3 gave almost identical results. The cap was formed in less than twelve hours, and by the middle of the second

If a very sweet wine is desired, as those of Andalusia and some of Catalonia, the moment the fermentation begins a certain amount of alcohol is added to the must, thus preventing the splitting up of the sugar and leaving to the wine in consequence its natural sweetness.

And nevertheless this wine, which contains all the elements necessary to fermentation, ferment, sugar, etc., never undergoes this change, since it always retains its sweetness.

In the same work of M. Duclaux that makes a perfectly clear summary of all the theories and all the experiments relative to fermentations, we find two other passages that corroborate and confirm our idea.

"Alcohol, which is the product of fermentations, is detrimental to all of them, but not in the same degree.

"*Certain fermentations cease when the proportion of alcohol formed is, say, two per cent or even less, after which they remain inactive no matter how large the quantity of sugar present. The others allow the formation of ten, twelve, and even fifteen per cent of alcohol, and these naturally are the beers most prized and sought after.*"

Here we have again a case in which fermentation has

day, the fermentations had reached their maximum, evolving from seventy to seventy-five bubbles of gas per minute. Finally, the fermentation was complete on the 14th of September when that in flask No. 1 had barely begun.

"These experiments prove that yeast of wine, when cultivated and added to the must, rapidly induces its fermentation, and that it may be completely effected at relatively low temperatures between 15° and 20° C. instead of from 30° to 35°." (*Sur la puissance de la levure de vin, cultivée.* Note by M. ALPH. ROMMIER, *Academy of Sciences*, 30th June, 1884.

been arrested by the presence of alcohol, which cannot be explained but by the action that we attribute to the leuco-maines on the microbes that have elaborated them.

In another passage on the same subject of beers, he says: "*From this moment it no longer ferments or very little. Nevertheless, it still contains sugar.*

"Why has not this sugar fermented, *since there is yet yeast?*

"*It is because this yeast has become weakened.*

"*A prolonged contact with carbonic acid is noxious to it, as we have seen.*"

In this case, it is the carbonic acid that produces the same effect, and this effect must be attributed to the same cause, as carbonic acid is also a leucomaine of the *mycoderma* that produces alcoholic fermentation.

Here we have three experiments in which the microbes that give rise to them are perfectly well known to us, and their leucomaines also, for these substances and these microbes have been long studied; now, in these three experiments, which are so much the more valuable on account of our more perfect knowledge of them, *we find the complete confirmation of our theory.*

PART THIRD.

EXPLANATION OF SOME PHENOMENA BY THIS THEORY.

EXPLANATION OF SOME PHENOMENA BY THIS THEORY.

CHAPTER I.

CRISES OF INFECTIOUS DISEASES.

A phenomenon characteristic of all infectious maladies is that of crisis.

In these disorders it is known beforehand that at the end of a certain length of time, one or two weeks for instance, the disease will produce a crisis with either a favorable or fatal termination.

If the sick person resists the crisis, his state improves daily, he recovers his forces, and finally is cured.

If, on the contrary, he is unable to resist the crisis, or does not retain sufficient strength to recover after passing it, he succumbs inevitably and dies.

The microbian theories, and what we have hitherto set forth, will likewise explain this phenomenon.

I demonstrate it by comparing these diseases to an alcoholic fermentation.

Observe what takes place in the production of beer.

"The alcohol produced by fermentations is an obstacle to heir further operation, but acts in different degrees on each one. Some are arrested when the proportion of alcohol formed reaches two per cent for instance, or even when the quantity is smaller, and then remain inactive, no matter what the amount of sugar still unchanged may be. Others withstand the presence in the fermentation fluid of ten, twelve, and even fifteen per cent of alcohol, and these naturally are those most prized and used." *

We observe that fermentation is produced and continues increasing till the microbes find themselves in contact with their leucomaines in the proportion of two, ten, twelve or fifteen per cent.

At this moment, either the life of the microbes or their reproduction is put an end to, leaving unchanged the sugar in the fluid, whatever its proportions.

What are the points of resemblance between fermentation and infectious disease ?

A microbe produces fermentation, and a microbe likewise is the cause of infectious disease.

In the first case, the microbe derives its life from the sugar.

In the interior of man the microbe lives at the cost of the blood and substances in the tissues.

In fermentation, when the alcohol attains the proportion before mentioned, the microbe remains inactive, and consequently the fermentation ceases.

In disease, when a crisis supervenes, can it not be, as in fermentation, that a sufficient number of leucomaines has been formed to arrest the life of the microbes ?

* *Le Microbe et la Maladie,* by E. Duclaux, page 82.

When this moment arrives, the sick person retains the elements not taken away by the microbes.

If these elements are yet in sufficient number so that the thread of life be not broken, the individual will return to his ordinary state of health; if, on the contrary, he has been deprived of them, he will die.

If our theory be not accepted, what explanation can be given of those numerous cases in which, after this crisis is passed, the sick persons have been cured without any remedy having been administered ?

If the action which in our opinion belongs to the leucomaines be not attributed to them, we would have to admit that in these diseases the microbes should live and multiply until the complete exhaustion of all the substances man is able to furnish them with for their nourishment; and as the total absence of these substances implies death, these diseases would all terminate fatally.

Experience, however, tells us that a large number of subjects recover without it being possible to attribute this favorable result to the action of medicines.

CHAPTER II.

By accepting this theory, phenomena are explained that formerly were inexplicable.

Why, for instance, should an epidemic of cholera last longer when less intense ?

And why should it be shorter when more intense ?

The reason is that the more intense it is and the more microbes there are, their life is just so much the more active, and consequently there must be a greater number of leucomaines exerting a baneful influence on these same microbes.

If, on the contrary, the epidemic is light, it is because there is a smaller number of microbes, which being distributed by the waters or other vehicles, can easily escape the action of their own leucomaines.

It is also easy, by means of this theory, to explain the fact, which seemed extraordinary, of a town where cholera has raged during one year being free from that scourge the next, while another one subject to the same atmospheric conditions, but not attacked the first year, is contaminated the second.

It ought naturally to be inferred that the first of these towns was more in danger than the second, as there would always be numerous germs in the first, while in the second there would be none.

The actual fact can only be explained by admitting that the poison that destroys the microbe is a product of the microbe itself.

The falsity of the idea of the attenuation of microbes is equally evident from all these facts.

This attenuation of microbes would lead us to believe that when an epidemic in a city has begun to decrease, it is because the microbe producing it has become attenuated, and consequently, if imported into another city, it ought to be mild in form. Very numerous well-proved facts are, however, in absolute disagreement with this opinion.

By the theory herein exposed, cholera must necessarily sooner or later disappear from Europe.

How then is it endemic in Asia? It is because in the East the putrefaction of dead bodies in the delta of the Ganges engenders the micro-organism of cholera which no putrefaction in Europe produces.*

* The comma bacillus, like every other organism, must follow the laws of vegetation, the same as the larger plants; it must reproduce and bring forth its like, and it cannot come from a vegetable belonging to another species, much less be the product of nothing. And as comma-bacilli are micro-organisms that do not reproduce in all countries, we must infer that the disease occasioned by them comes precisely from the spot where it is born spontaneously. We cannot admit the supposition, nevertheless made by serious persons, that cholera was engendered spontaneously in the delta of the Nile, and in British East India; neither can we accept that cholera could have presented itself in Europe before the importation of the comma-bacillus. (KOCH, *Imperial Council of Berlin*, sitting of 26th July, 1884.)

There exists in the southern countries of India, in the south of

It is these contingents of putrefaction that cause the endemic state of cholera is Asia.*

The same thing happens in Europe with typhus or typhoid fever, which is produced by the decay of animal matters in the waters of sewers, etc., and it is this that always gives a new contingent of microbes that produce this disease; and this is why in Europe typhus has the double character of being both endemic and epidemic, as happens with cholera in Asia.

Bengal, a large surface of alluvium grounds bathed by the numerous deltas of the Ganges.

In these swamps, where the detritus of organic matter in numberless quantities has been accumulating for centuries, and where a continuous high temperature maintains incessant fermentation, a special fauna and flora must have grown. Among other beings natural to this region, we must rank the comma-bacillus. As in all other parts, the circumstances of medium have created species strictly indigenous; the schizomycelium of cholera finds nowhere else the conditions necessary for its perpetuation. (VAN ERMENGEN.)

Contagious cholera never breaks out spontaneously in Europe; it is always imported from abroad. So far it has always come from Hindostan. (VAN ERMENGEN.)

* The regions of Southern Bengal are frequently inundated; the people live huddled together in the utmost degree of squalor and uncleanliness; while the stagnant waters serve for the most antihygienic purposes. For this reason cholera reigns there in an endemic state. (VAN ERMENGEN.)

CHAPTER III.

By this theory we can likewise explain the immunity with which poison may be taken, acquired by accustoming one's self to its use and increasing progressively the quantity up to mortal doses.

For this purpose we must distinguish poisons the cause of which is a microbe, and those in which the presence of none such can be admitted.

In the first case, i. e., when the poison is a substance

---

* *Poison:* a generic name for all substances that, introduced into the animal system by cutaneous absorption, the lungs in the act of breathing, or the digestive channels, act harmfully on the tissues of the organs in such a way as to put life in danger or to cause death in a very short time. (E. LITTRÉ.)

On account of the very extensive sense given by M. Littré to the word poison, we may observe that if every poisoning by microbes is not what would be called an infectious disease, still it is no less true that all infectious maladies are comprised under the head of poisonings caused by the introduction into the organisms of pathogenic microbes. For this reason the present chapter, that treats on the tolerance of microbe-containing poisons, explains how, during an epidemic, certain individuals escape from being attacked without, however, having contracted the disease or having been vaccinated. The absence of this sort of natural vaccination through having been accustomed to the poison it produces, explains how an epidemic is much more to be dreaded by persons entering a contaminated city coming from a healthy region. (THE AUTHOR.)

containing microbes which, on being introduced into the organism, grow therein, disturbing its functions, the explanation is as follows:*

It is known that it is necessary to begin by giving to the person who is to be accustomed to poison, a very small quantity of it, which experience has proved to be harmless to him who absorbs it.

Let us suppose that this quantity contains five microbes; these microbes introduced into the organism will live and die there, leaving behind five leucomaines.

The next day a quantity of poison containing eight microbes will be introduced, which quantity we also know is unable to produce any disturbance.

Of these eight microbes, five very probably will be killed by the leucomaines of the five previously introduced; the remaining three will live and produce three leucomaines: $5 + 3 = 8$ leucomaines.

If on the following day a quantity be introduced containing eight microbes, the effect will be null, as these eight microbes will be killed by the eight leucomaines elaborated by those previously introduced.

If, instead of a quantity containing eight microbes, one with thirteen be absorbed, as the organism already contained eight leucomaines, the effect produced will be only that of five microbes, and would be the same as in the first

---

* Very possibly the poisonous property of some articles of food that have undergone putrefaction, or some unknown kind of fermentation, is caused by some ferment, the product of micro-organisms (sausage poisoning, poisoning by bad fish and other articles). (DR. E. KLEIN, Micro-organisms and Disease, page 233.)

case, in which, as we know, no important disturbances are produced.*

This is how no effects are felt when, by habit, large quantities of poisons can be absorbed. The conditions are not the same for one who takes a large dose which is fatal and another who can take the same amount without feeling its effects.

The organism of the former contained no antidote, whereas in the latter it was already elaborated beforehand.

For poisons whose action cannot be attributed to micro-organisms, the explanation is also very simple.

In order that the reader may better accept my interpretation, I here transcribe the interesting and beautiful experiment of M. Raulin.

M. Raulin has made cultivations of a vegetable species; the *aspergillus niger*, and studied the different crops produced, according to the nourishment given to it and the substances most inimical to it.

The aspergillus niger belongs to the group of the mucedineæ, the most known type of which is common mould, and which are composed of a radicular system, called *my-*

---

*If we make use of figures, it is in order that our idea may be more easily grasped. If the microbe multiplies, there will always be the same proportion between the number of seeds sown and that of the amount of crop. If one hundred grains of wheat are gathered when ten are sown, the crop yielded by five grains will only be half of that in the former case.

The proportion of the quantity being always the same, our interpretation will be admitted under this respect. (Note by the AUTHOR.)

celium, living in the depths of the nourishing medium and of fruit-bearing organs, formed generally by a small column rising in the air bearing the fruit or spores.

The spores sown on favorable soil soon give off *branches of mycelian tubes*, the interlacing of which forms a thick, white layer.

This aspergillus grows very well on bread dampened with vinegar, on juice and slices of lemon, and in general on fruits and acid fluids.

M. Raulin has succeeded in constituting a medium favorable to the growth of this aspergillus, thus permitting him to make some interesting experiments.

The fluid, known as Raulin's fluid, has the following composition:

Water, .	1,500	gr.
Sugar candy, .	70	"
Tartaric acid, . .	4	"
Nitrate of ammonium, .	4	"
Phosphate of ammonium, .	0.6	"
Carbonate of potassium,	0.6	"
Carbonate of magnesium, .	0.4	"
Sulphate of ammonium, .	0.25	"
Sulphate of zinc,	0.07	"
Sulphate of iron, .	0.07	"
Silicate of potassium, .	0.07	"

To these elements must be added the oxygen of the air which is consumed in large quantities by the plant. It is likewise necessary to keep the fluid at a temperature of about 35° C. (95° F.) in a damp air renewed at convenient times.

"If when all these conditions are present, the surface of the fluid be planted with spores of the vegetable, at the end of twenty-four hours a whitish membrane is seen to form and cover the fluid. This is the mycelium of the plant. Fructification begins on the following day. At the end of three days, the cycle of vegetation is complete.

"As it is of interest to obtain the weight of the maximum crop for a given amount of sugar, we will employ these residues for the formation of new tissues. For this object, the plant formed is taken away, and spores are again sown in the remaining fluid. Three days after, a new crop is obtained somewhat weaker than the first.

"These two plants taken together are equivalent to twenty-five grammes of the plant weighed in dry air, and the nourishing fluid is then totally exhausted.

"With these elements of success, let us try to solve the problem set down in the beginning. Let us see, for instance, what is the measure of the usefulness of potassium in the fluid. For this object, let us make the plant live in two similar basins, one having Raulin's fluid complete, the other this fluid without potassium. In the first case, the result, as in ordinary cases, will be twenty-five grammes of plant. In the other only one gramme. The crop falls therefore to one-twenty-fifth of what it was. It falls to one-two-hundredth if phosphoric acid be suppressed; to one one-hundred-and-fiftieth when ammonium is suppressed. . . . . The suppression of zinc reduces the amount collected to one-tenth of what it was in the normal fluid, that is to say, it decreases from twenty-five grammes to two and a half. Was it to be suspected that zinc constituted a physiological element of so much importance ? The quantity of sulphate of zinc employed was seven centigrammes containing only thirty-two milligrammes of zinc. The action of this extremely small quantity of metal is, however, sufficient to increase the amount of the crop in twenty-two and a half grammes; in other words, it allows the formation of seven hundred times its weight in the plant.

"Is this not indeed singular?

"Does it not become even more so when we bear in mind that the plant, which is so sensitive to the action of zinc, must absorb it in a liquid in which it is diluted in the homœopathic dose of one-one-fifty-thousandth? . . . .

"If, as we have just seen, the aspergillus is extremely sensitive to the action of elements necessary to it, it is still more so to that of those which are prejudicial to it. If to the nourishing fluid one-sixteen-hundred-thousandth ($\frac{1}{1600000}$) of nitrate of silver be added, the vegetation is abruptly arrested. It cannot even begin in a silver receptacle, although it be impossible for chemical analysis to show that the least part of the substance of the receptacle has become dissolved in the fluid. But the plant, much more sensitive than the chemical reagents, which, however, are very much so as regards salts of silver, denounces, by refusing to grow, the presence of the poisonous substance. One-five-hundred-thousandth ($\frac{1}{500000}$) of corrosive sublimate has the same effect, so have one-eight-thousandth of bichloride of platinum and one-two-hundred-and-fortieth of sulphate of copper. . . .

"One more experimental fact remains to be pointed out. The plant not containing green matter, one may be surprised to see iron among the number of its nutritive elements. The suppression of this metal produces, however, effects similar to those caused by the suppression of zinc. The introduction of one gramme of iron into the nutritive medium increases the amount of plant eight hundred fold.

"In spite of this resemblance, the *role* of zinc and that of iron are entirely distinct. The zinc enters the plant as a constituent element of its tissues. The only use for the iron seems to be its action on a poison secreted by the plant which it destroys as soon as formed. If this poison were permitted to accumulate in the fluid, it would finally kill the plant; it is one of those excretions that all living bodies produce, and which they must rid themselves of at any cost. Iron renders this service to the aspergillus. Zinc is a physiological aliment; iron, a physiological antidote." *

We have seen the effect of mineral substances on the vegetation of aspergillus niger. Now, in order to arrive at our conclusion, viz., the explanation of the law of toleration of poisons that are not microbes, it is necessary to accept the hypothesis of the existence in the organism of germs or microbes.

* E. DUCLAUX, *Le Microbe et la Maladie*, Chapter IV.

† The following are some of the conclusions with which M. Bechamp finishes a memoir presented to the Academy of Medicine, the 20th of April, 1886:

"1st. The interior of living bodies is not something passive similar to a vessel filled with fermentable matters; and originally there do not exist morbid germs in the air, the water, and the earth.

"2d. The living organism lives in all its parts, not on account occult properties, but rather because being formed by anatomical elements living *per se* . . . which are the microzymas.

"3d. The organism does not contain germs of attenuated microbes either latent or apparent, strange to it. . . . But the microzymæ of these different regions and organs become in certain cases what has been improperly termed microbes.

This hypothesis can be admitted without difficulty, as the greater part of micrologists have proved the existence of germs or of microbes in the animal organism. The explanation from this point ahead is similar to that for the first case: the poison introduced into the organism _acts by occasioning the birth of germs, or by increasing the crop of microbes the presence of which we have admitted.*

"Still more : as I knew the symptoms, always complicated, of a poisoning by arsenic, I intoxicated animals with this substance and performed their autopsy after death. I discovered large quantities of bacteria, but no comma bacilli." (Dr. Koch, Session of the Imperial Council of Berlin, 26th July, 1884.)

A small quantity of poison acts on a small number of microbes, and the toxic effect is due to the action of these microbes as in the first case. These microbes leave behind their leucomaines. A larger quantity of poison develops a larger number of microbes which, by their own leucomaines, as well as by those of the microbes that preceded

"4th. The living body is not refractory to the introduction of micro-organisms from outside." (BÉCHAMP, *Bulletin de l'Académie de Médecine*, Session of 20th April, 1886, page 577.)

The coexistence of the comma bacillus and the choleric process may be explained by supposing that the choleric process so modifies the vital condition of the intestine that one of the numerous species of bacteria, normally present in the intestine, is changed into comma bacillus, etc. (*Recherches sur le microbe du cholera asiatique*, by Doctor E. VAN ERMENGEN.

* An experiment made by Koch, in his researches on the comma bacillus of cholera, seems to uphold the idea of the growth of the microbes due to the presence of poisons, and on which we have based our explanation of the action of these latter.

them, would, after a certain time, perish, leaving also their leucomaines.

The sum of the leucomaines of the first two doses will destroy in part or altogether the toxic action of the third dose, and so on.

By means of the experiment of M. Raulin, we can also explain the law of tolerance of poisons. Let us suppose the existence in the animal system of germs of aspergillus, and let us introduce as a poison Raulin's fluid deprived of iron, on account of the action of this substance on the leucomaines which we are in search of.

This done, let us admit that the crop of aspergillus deprived of iron be in a quantity of liquid equal to that before mentioned (two grammes and a half).

Let us further suppose that there is an unlimited number of germs in the organism and, consequently, that the crop depends on the quantity of nourishing fluid as in M. Raulin's experiment; and that the aspergillus elaborates a weight of substances of leucomaines equal to that of the crop of this plant.

These points accepted, let us introduce in the organism, where we have supposed the existence of germs of aspergillus, half the quantity of fluid that has served M. Raulin as a type for his calculations; we have a crop one-half smaller, thus:

FIRST DOSE.

Nourishing fluid, . 789.99 Crop of

Crop of leucomaines, 1.25 Aspergillus, . . . 1.25

Since these 789.99 of fluid give a maximum yield of 1.25

aspergillus and 1.25 of leucomaines, and that after producing this crop the fluid remains sterile, let us admit that 1.25 of leucomaines sterilize 789.99 of fluid.

This hypothesis being accepted, let us see what passes with the second dose.

SECOND DOSE.

As a second dose we will employ 1,579.990: As we already have 1.25 of leucomaines, and as we have just said that these 1.25 sterilize 789.99 of liquid, we must take away from the amount of fresh fluid introduced what will be sterilized immediately by the presence of leucomaines.

Nourishing fluid,	1,579.990	Growth of		
do. sterilized,	789.995	Aspergillus,	. . .	1.25
	————	Production		
	789.995	of leucomaines,	.	1.25

Leucomaines produced:

From the first dose,	.	.	.	.	1.25
From the second dose,	.	.		.	1.25
				———
				2.50

THIRD DOSE.

For this dose we will introduce in the system 2,369.985 of fluid, of which 1,579.990 will be sterilized immediately by the 2.50 of leucomaines already present.

Nourishing fluid,	2,369.985	Aspergillus		
do. sterilized,	1,579.990	produced,	. .	1.25
	————	Leucomaines,	. .	1.25
	789.995			

Production of leucomaines:

From the first dose, .	. 1.25
From the second dose, .	1.25
From the third dose, .	. 1.25
	———
	3.75

By these calculations we can see that in the second or third doses the amount of aspergillus has been equal to that of the first dose, in spite of the nourishing fluid being double and triple that of the first.

Thus we see how, according to our theory, we can explain the necessity of increasing the doses of poison in order to sustain its toxic or therapeutic action.

CHAPTER IV.

EXPLANATION OF SEVERAL OTHER PHENOMENA BY DIFFERENT AUTHORS.

On the appearance of the first edition of the present work, many critics and scientific men reported it in periodicals, reviews and academies, and some not only gave their opinion of it, but, convinced of the truth of the theory therein set forth, perceived that by its means certain phenomena were easily explained for which till then no plausible explanation had been given.

The labors of these scientists are in reality a continuation of that begun by myself in this part of my work, as a proof of my theory.

It seems to me, therefore, very much in place to add, in the present chapter, the extracts of the various scientific labors I refer to, and which increase the stock of phenomena already explained by me.

CHANCROID.—The important review, *Lyon Médical*, official organ of the Society of Medicine and Medical Sciences, published in its issue of October 31st, 1886, an article dedicated to the examination of my theory, signed with the initials P. D.

These initials and the elegant style of the article reveal the name of a well-known scientist, author of several works which have gained for him the enviable fame of a profound physician and eminent writer.

This author, in the article already referred to, writes as follows regarding the terrible ulcer known as *chancroid*.

"Coming under our special domain, we have a little disease, the evolution and, principally, the termination of which has openly defied the sagacity of physicians. *Chancroid* (simple chancre) is an ulcer contagious in the highest degree, that increases by the unceasing spontaneous inoculation from its circumference. But, why is this labor arrested? How is it that, while the pus of this ulcer still continues contagious for every other region, there arrives a time when it ceases to be so for its immediate vicinity? This very serious question, requiring an urgent reply, was answered evasively by saying that it was owing to a cause as mysterious, but as real, as that by which the Deity contained the sea when He said, '*Non procedes amplius.*' At present, without soaring so high, but not on that account renouncing the teachings of history, we may say that the ulcer is circumscribed by a process similar to that suggested by patriotism to the Russians in Moscow; namely, by making an uninhabitable circle around the conqueror."

BABES' PLATES.—The young and skilled physicians, Drs. Carreras,* known by their works on microbiology, referring to my theory in an article written in Davos Platz

---

* One of them, Dr. Louis, died very recently. His loss has been deeply felt, not only by his friends, but likewise by true lovers of science, to which he applied himself with great tact and success.

(Switzerland), and addressed to the *Barcelona Review of Medical Sciences*, in which it appeared on the 10th of February, 1887, made the following remarks explaining the phenomenon observed by Babes.

"Even in the pathogenic microbes we also observe similar facts. For this object, following Babes' example, put in a small glass cell, capable of being hermetically closed with a cover-glass, a layer of agar-agar or gelatin conveniently sterilized. With a platinum thread, impregnated with microbes of anthrax, cholera, or other similar disease, let a large circumference be drawn and the plate then be placed in the incubator. At the end of one or two weeks or a month, when the entire large circumference has produced a good growth, let parallel arcs be drawn with platinum thread impregnated with the same or different microbes. It will be seen that almost always the microbes of the first circle hinder partially or completely the germination of microbes of a similar nature sown later on. Thus, making the large circumference with the cholera bacillus, and eight days after drawing parallel lines with the same bacillus, the growth takes place very slowly; and if the second lines be drawn fifteen days after the first, there is hardly any growth whatever. The same phenomenon is observed with the bacillus of anthrax, the microbe of blue pus, the *staphylococcus aureus*, and many others. Some chromogenic microbes even lose their distinctive color. Planting parallel lines of *staphylococcus aureus* six days after making the large circumference, there is an exceedingly small growth with scarcely any color. This antagonism would, at first sight, seem to admit being explained

by the exhaustion of the soil; but if it is borne in mind that
the microbe that forms the first circle goes slowly invading
the entire mass of gelatin, and therefore finds sufficient
elements of nutrition, the lack of growth in the parallel
lines cannot be explained by the want of nutritious elements.

"The most probable explanation is that the microbes of
the first circumference give rise to leucomaines that are
diffused in the periphery. As a curious example of this
diffusion, we remember having observed in a tube of gelatin somewhat cloudy the formation of two small colonies
of microbes. In their vicinity the gelatin became perfectly transparent in a large space, owing to the diffusion
of the leucomaines. Thus, when the parallel lines before
mentioned are drawn, the microbes they contain do not
thrive, or do so with difficulty, on account of being in contact with an excess of toxic leucomaines; as, besides those
engendered by themselves, they receive also those that are
diffused from the large circumference."

ABRAHAM COLLES' LAW AND OTHER PHENOMENA.—At
the opening of the session for 1888 of the Barcelona Scho-
lastic Medical Athenæum, the president of that body, Dr.
Felipe Proubasta, read a very learned and scientific paper
on the "*Theories of Immunity*," from which, on account
of their reference to the theory of *Leucomaines*, we copy
the following extracts:

". . . The same explanation given in the *Lyon Medical*
for the soft chancre may be used for every local infectious

process when the lymphatic circulation does not carry off
the micro-organism to new grounds which, not having
suffered from its havoc, may become a new theatre for its
devastation. To make this proposition clear, it will be sufficient for me to lay before you a case for which, up to the
present, no explanation has been given, but which is easily
understood if we admit the theory of *immunity through
leucomaines.* You all know that from time immemorial
motion has been considered the worst poison for fungous
arthritis; so much so that professors of clinic have endeavored to attenuate the morbific process by the use of immov-
able bandages and apparatus in the belief that, if by their
means ankylosis could be established, the member, and
even the individual, in the greater number of cases could
be considered saved. In a word, it is an axiom in surgical
pathology that the best drug for white swelling in the beginning is rest. Now, observe in what a simple manner
we can explain the cure of white swelling in these circumstances with this theory.

"Let us suppose that Koch's tubercular bacilli have
entered a joint; their leucomaines would be produced, and
those beings would finally perish from contact with these
products of their nutrition, like the inhabitants of Sodom
by the fire brought on by their sins, unless a family of a
microscopical Lot, flying from the wrath of the flavus
through the lymphatic current, reproduce the disease in
another spot near or remote. But the lymphatic current,
in no place rapid, is especially torpid in the epiphyses of
bones where the tubercular swellings are formed, probably
as the continuation of a synovial exudate; the reason is
that nature counted on the powerful aid that articular

movements would lend to the lymphatic circulation. Suppress these movements and the lymphatic current in this place will be almost negative; do the same in a joint with a restricted tubercular process, and the bacilli, condemned to quietude in one place, will die by the poisoning of the surrounding medium with their leucomaines.

" Many other examples I could mention with a similar explanation; the same considerations could be made in regard to carbuncle, erysipelas, and other local processes. However, I do not wish to pass over in silence a fact in support of this theory which gives a plausible explanation of it; a fact, the cause of which is obscure, and which, though considered as a scientific monstrosity, is universally admitted, and has even been raised to a law. We refer to a phenomenon that may occur, during pregnancy, to the mother and to the fœtus, when the former cohabits with a syphilitic individual.

"Take the case of such a person having intercourse with a healthy woman in a state of pregnancy. One of two things may happen; either both the mother and the fœtus may be contaminated or one of them only. In this latter case, it may be the mother or it may be the fœtus that acquires syphilis.

" If it is the child, the mother remains exempt from the disease, and she may with impunity nurse at her breasts the being she bore in her womb, even though it have ulcers or mucous patches in its mouth. This fact, apparently so exceptional, was, however, laid down as a law in 1844 by Abraham Colles, and in spite of the objections made to it in the beginning, and of the exceptions pretended to have been found by Amilcare Ricordi in his treatise *Sifilide da Allatamento*, it was and has been accepted by all.

"No one up to the present has been able to account for this law of Colles, and Robin must have had it in mind when, on mentioning what occurs to the mother and child in presence of an infective state, he declares that there is no possible explanation of the phenomena observed.

"Mr. Güell's theory of immunity throws on this dark point so much light, that for me the problem is solved.

"You know, indeed, that for the fact to occur there must be a certain degree of independence between the fœtus and its mother in their placentary relations—an independence that will make it impossible for the syphilitic bacillus to cross the placentary barrier; but if the organism, cause of the disease, cannot enter the current of circulation of the mother, we may, however, easily conceive the ingress into it of the leucomaines of this micro-organism, bestowing thereby on the mother the immunity before referred to, as the diffusibility of these leucomaines is admirably adapted to it.

"In my opinion, the same explanation can be given for Profeta's law, viz.: the fact that a child born of a syphilitic mother, without having contracted the contagion within the womb, has an immunity from this disease.

Your own clear judgment will readily perceive the revolution that the admission of this theory would produce in the field of therapeutics should new facts not come, as I do not believe they will, to destroy or essentially modify it, and it be accepted completely. The homœopathic principle would become the base of medication in infectious diseases, and physicians would not hesitate to introduce the leucomaines into the human system before a crisis is produced by its saturation with microbes alone. We can easily understand that this should be done, as the system is better disposed, at the beginning of an infection, to resist the leucomainic poisoning than later on, when fever has wasted the greater part of the radical organic forces. The inoculations might even be made with substances unmixed with germs, which might either be the leucomaines or substances with a similar a tonic constitution and endowed with like properties.

" And do not believe, gentlemen, that this is an indication based entirely on a theoretical conception. Two antecedents exist in support of this view that I do not wish to leave unmentioned before proceeding to review other theories of immunity.

" *First fact*—You all know that at present it is generally admitted that the surest remedy for any infection would be to find a vaccine which having a period of incubation much shorter than the disease should preserve the system from the effects of this latter. Unfortunately, this can only be applied in a very small number of cases, of which rabies is one. In small-pox it is only feasible at the very beginning of the disease, performing the vaccination in the ordinary way following the advice of the American Dr. Driai. But when it is too late to proceed thus, we can still have recourse to the intensive model, substituting the three prickings on each arm at one sitting with a smaller number repeated for two, three, or more days ; otherwise both diseases develop together independent of each other."

Now, observe how I explain this method with the theory I am now examining.

We will suppose a man vaccinated in a state of health. The vaccine will have produced a certain quantity of leucomaines, say l, sufficient to counteract a given number I of variolic microbes. If the disease be already in an advanced state, the I microbes will have increased to say m I; if in these circumstances vaccination be performed by the ordinary method, the most that will be produced will be $\frac{1}{4}$ leucomaines, and even to reach this number a certain number of days must elapse. This amount of leucomaines, $\frac{1}{4}$ will be powerless to counteract the infection of m. I microbes unless the disease be taken at its outset. But if a much greater quantity of micro-organisms of the vaccine be inoculated in five or six different times by the intensive method, in the cellular tissue there will be formed, even without sufficient time having passed for the vaccine disease to manifest itself, $m'l$ leucomaines sufficient to check the effects of m. I variolic microbes. In a word, the effect is produced, not by the fact of the sick person having suffered from the vaccine malady, but by the $m'l$ leucomaines engendered by the micro-organisms introduced with the lancet into the cellular tissue.

Another fact.—M. Payraud, in a note presented to the Academy of Medicine by Brown-Séquard, declares that the injection of the essence of tansy into the cellular tissue of animals susceptible to anthrax produces symptoms resembling rabies, and preserves them from this disease. For this scientist—and I quite agree with him—this is owing to the fact that this substance has an atonic constitution similar to that of the leucomaines produced by the hydrophobic virus, the presence of which in the system gives immunity.

FINAL OBSERVATION.

The actual state of science, in the opinion of some very learned men, is still as obscure as previously.

Virchow has said in a speech that "the discovery of microbes has only made the difficulty recede without solving it; the struggle of life and death, of the organism against disease, has become the battle of cells against bacteria; the ground is more circumscribed, but the details of the combat are still a mystery to us."

We believe, however, that science has thrown a great deal of light on these questions by the grand discovery of microbes, that must necessarily have brought us much nearer to the solution, as, with one step, we have entered into a whole new world, that of the infinitely small and at the same time infinitely powerful.

In infectious maladies, we no longer assist at the incomprehensible struggle of life and death; the struggle is between two beings having similar wants.

This struggle, therefore, presents itself on a ground much better known, and in conditions almost equal; for if the organized beings whose existence has been so long known to us are much larger, the infinitely small beings are infinitely more numerous.

That there are still many obscure points no one doubts. There are even contradictions between the experiments that have been made, as every one knows; but no one must wonder at it, as we are only at the beginning of micrological sciences. This circumstance should only teach us not to accept as indisputable all the experimental facts, principally those not in accordance with general laws the truth of which is known to us.

On looking for materials with which to support and develop the work now finishing, I have come across many experimental facts not in accordance with my idea..

I have not, however, receded before such facts, for a theory should not be abandoned simply because some experimental facts are contrary to it, if it has the power of explaining clearly other experiments and a large number of natural phenomena that till now had not been explained.

Among the experiments in opposition to what I have just said, the most important is that of M. Pasteur in 1880. But in a note sent to the Academy of Sciences the 28th of October, 1885,* he declares that this experiment must be repeated, as he has foreseen, with regard to the inoculations

---

* " Still another interpretation can be given of the new method, an interpretation certainly very strange at first sight, but which deserves all our attention, because it is in harmony with certain results already known, that phenomena of life present us among the lower beings, principally among several pathogenic microbes.

" Many microbes seem to give rise in their cultures to matters detrimental to their growth. In the year 1880, I have instituted researches in order to establish the fact that the microbe of fowl-cholera produces a sort of poison for this microbe

" I did not succeed in proving that such a substance existed, but at present I believe these experiments should be performed anew, and for my part, I would not fail to operate in pure carbonic acid." (PASTEUR, *Comptes rendus* of the Academy of Sciences, Vol. XV., 1880.)

of the virus of rabies, an explanation that would be entirely in accord with our theory.

It is with the hope that this theory will be recognized as *true*, and consequently that it may render some benefits to mankind, that we deliver it to the public in general and to men of science in particular. To these latter, we would say, as in olden times did Chremes, the personage of Terence, to his interlocutor Menedemus: "Take what I tell you either as an advice I give you, or as instructions I demand from you." *

* TERENCE, *Hoautontuorumenos*, Act I., Scene I., verse 78.

REPLY TO THE OBJECTIONS RAISED AGAINST IMMUNITY THROUGH LEUCOMAINES.

REPLY TO THE OBJECTIONS

RAISED AGAINST

IMMUNITY THROUGH LEUCOMAINES.

At the end of a critical article on the first edition of this work, Mr. Zaborowski thus expressed himself:

" A theory of immunity ought to explain to us at the same time the natural immunity of Algerine sheep from anthrax and of negroes against yellow fever, as well as that acquired by preserva tive inoculations." *

As regards this observation, we must remark: That every law corresponds to a certain order of phenomena, and that, in the case mentioned above, the so-styled natural immunity corresponds to an order of phenomena entirely different from that we have undertaken to explain, and in reality distinct from that which comprises the non-recurrence of infectious diseases and, consequently, vaccinations.

In order to render this statement clearer, we must explain what is the true idea of immunity as it is at present understood in regard to the animal organisms and parasitary maladies.

In these latter, the system is not an actor, but plays a passive part. The agent or actor is a microbe of such and

* *La Justice*, Paris, 7th October, 1886.

such a disease, that on entering the system for the first time proliferates there, that is to say, germinates, grows, and multiplies. But, on penetrating for the second time, the same thing does not happen.

On penetrating for the second time, the microbe remains powerless, does not reproduce, or dies. This is the phenomenon that nature presents us to which the name of immunity has been given.

Why does this microbe, on penetrating for the second time, perish, if the first time and in the same medium it thrived ? This is the true problem to be solved, and which we believe we have succeeded in doing: thus presented in its true light, we believe there is no possible doubt.

If a microbe, A or B, be introduced into a recipient having a temperature say of 200° C., this microbe will die. Would it be logical to comprise this phenomenon under the same head as that just mentioned ? In this case, the microbe dies on penetrating for the first time into the receiving medium, while in the former, which is the true problem, the basis is precisely contrary; that is to say, the first time the microbe thrives, but not the second.

Therefore, the so-called natural immunity of Algerine sheep from anthrax does not correspond to the series of phenomena treated of in this work.

Is it possible for leucomaines to persist in the system all the time that immunity exists, which, in some cases, is very long?

Such is the question, or more properly the objection, that some present to my theory.*

* *La Justice*, Paris, 7th October, 1886, and others.

Among the substances penetrating the system, some act physiologically, others prophylactically, others pathologically, while some exert no action whatever, or one that is unknown.

The first class, viz., those that enter in order to fulfil some object in the state of health, such as those destined to nutrition, cannot remain long in the system in the same state in which they penetrated, since, in order to fill the vacancies that occur in the system, they have to undergo decompositions and transformations under the influence of numerous internal agents, being changed and converted into the elements that constitute our organism in a healthy tate.

With the exception of these, foreign bodies or substances may, in our opinion, remain for a longer or shorter period within the system. Some there are, the presence and pathological action of which persist throughout life. This we see, for instance, in some cases of poisoning by mercury, lead, or arsenic.

Other bodies remain inactive, *v. g.*, a silver wire, the paint on the bodies of Indians, and substances used for tattooing.

All that can be said *a priori* is, that bodies destined to fill a physiological need cannot persist in the organism in the state in which they penetrate; but those that are not in this case may remain unchanged for an indefinite space of time, as proved by numerous instances.

Leucomaines not being among the former, there is no reason to doubt the probability of their existence in the system during all the time that immunity lasts.

APPENDIX.

APPENDIX.

NOTE I.

MY DEAR M. DUCLAUX:—

§ 2.

What idea can be formed regarding the cause of immunity from rabies, after being bitten, by the prophylactic method? The first thought offering itself, is the supposition that the permanence of the rabic medullæ in dry air, of the temperature of 23° to 25° Centigr., gradually diminishes the virulence of these medullæ, until it is entirely destroyed. This naturally leads us to the belief that this method rests on the employment of virus which in the first instance is without appreciable virulence, becoming afterwards feeble, and gradually stronger. Notwithstanding the limitations in this respect, which I formulated in my communication to the Academy of Sciences, on 26th October, 1885, this explanation seems to have been generally accepted, and we find it everywhere expressed. We must confess that it has in its favor all the probabilities, as the rabic medullæ, put in desiccation at 23° to 25°, and inoculated to rabbits by trepannation, communicate to them the rabies, after a lapse of inoculation, at variance with the time of exposition to the dry air, and that after a fortnight of desiccation, the medullæ generally are no longer virulent. In the application of the theory, the non-virulent medullæ are succeeded by medullæ which appear progressively virulent. But experience demonstrates, as it seems, that these delays in the time of incubation are the effect of impoverishment in the quantity of virulence. And really, if you take again virus from rabbits of retarded time of incubation, even if delayed for a whole month, you will constantly and immediately obtain again

rabies of seven days' incubation, if inoculated by trepannation to fresh rabbits.   It might be objected to the hypothesis
propounded by me, that the carbunculous vaccine resumes
its virulence, if it causes accidentally the death of a sheep
or a cow.   It might also be objected that the heated carbunculous bacteridia, which becomes vaccinable at 55°, resumes its virulence by a simple cultivation.   Occasion can
be found to try the reproduction of the refractory state by
very small quantities of rabic virus, daily increasing in
quantity.   Yet, as regards the carbuncle, one cannot successfully vaccinate by this method.   The sheep will die
more slowly, but still they die, and will not become refractory.   After all we do not lose sight of the very original
and fruitful theory of Mr. Metschnikoff.   The vaccine substance, if it exists, will it be found in the dead microbes?

The rule, laid down above, is absolute.   In the application of the method, we would therefore not have to deal
with feeble virus, becoming gradually stronger.   The virulence would always be the same, and would only obey the
law of the variable lapse of duration by quantities, becoming gradually smaller, of a virus which would not change.

The facts, however, agree better with the idea of a vaccine matter, associated with the rabic microbe, and the latter retaining its own virulence unimpaired, in all medullæ
in desiccation, but undergoing in the same a progressive
destruction, quicker than the vaccine matter.   This opinion will be still further confirmed by the following facts:
Every method of inoculation of the rabies, the inoculation
of the virus underneath the dura-mater always excepted,
occasions a refractory state of the rabies, without any appearance of attenuated rabical malady.   I could quote innumerable examples of this fact, but will limit myself to
only a few.

On the 12th February, 1885, with the macerated medulla.
diluted in sterilized broth, of a street dog, which died of
violent rabies at the College of Alford, six young dogs were
inoculated, each one with a full Pravaz syringe, underneath the abdominal skin.   On the 6th March, one of the
six dogs was attacked by violent rabies, with pronounced
rabical barking.   On the 24th March, the remaining five dogs
were still doing well, and were inoculated again, this time
by the operation of trepanning, and with virus derived
from violent rabies from the street.   This new inoculation
resulted in three dogs attacked by rabies, the 4th, 5th, and
10th April, and two refractory dogs, which consequently

owed their refractory condition to the subcutaneous inoculation of 12th February.

On 23d July, 1886, seven young dogs were inoculated underneath the abdominal skin, each by one Pravaz syringe, filled with the medulla, diluted in sterilized broth, from a rabbit of the forty-seventh passage from rabbit to rabbit, the first rabbit of the series having received virus from a rabid street dog by trepanning. On the 5th August following, two of the seven dogs were attacked by paralytic rabies, lying down, and without inclination to bite or bark. On the 6th August the rabic paralysis commenced on the third dog, the 7th August on the fourth, the 10th August on the fifth, and the 25th August on the sixth. On the contrary, the seventh dog showed no sign of malady, either in August or September. To prove if he had become refractory in consequence of the inoculation of 23d July, he was inoculated by trepanning with virus from a rabid street-dog, but he showed no signs of uneasiness in the following months. Consequently he had become refractory.

On the 31st July, seven other young dogs were inoculated underneath the abdominal skin, each by a Pravaz syringe, containing the medulla of a rabid street-dog, macerated in sterilized liquid. Five of these dogs were attacked by rabies; the first on the 17th of August, by snapping hydrophobia with paralysis of the hind quarters; the second, on the 19th August; the third, fourth, and fifth on 28th August and 3d September, all four with paralytic rabies. There remained two in good health at the end of September, at which time they were again inoculated, by trepanning, with the medulla of a rabid street-dog. During the following months their health was perfect, and consequently they had been made refractory by the inoculation of 31st July.

On 23d January, 1885, six young dogs were inoculated underneath the abdominal skin, each with half a Pravaz syringe of the medulla, macerated in sterilized liquid, from the sixty-sixth passage from rabbit to rabbit. Five of these dogs were attacked with paralytic rabies after eleven, twelve, and thirteen days from the time of inoculation. One resisted and proved himself refractory, in consequence of the inoculation of 23d January.

On 13th July, 1886, seven young dogs were inoculated beneath the abdominal skin, each with two Pravaz syringes, filled with a medulla, macerated in sterilized liquid, from the one hundred and eighteenth passage from rabbit to rabbit.

On the 20th July one of these dogs was attacked with paralytic rabies. He was lying down paralyzed, snapping at a stick presented to him. The other six dogs resisted, and suffered afterwards an inoculation, as a trial, by means of trepanning, with the medulla of a rabid street-dog. Four of these dogs proved themselves refractory, and were so, through the effect of their inoculation of 13th July. The other two were attacked with paralytic rabies, but only after twenty-seven and twenty-eight days from the time of trepanning. This latter fact goes to prove that their inoculation of 13th July had not made them entirely refractory, but it proves also that they were nevertheless partially vaccinated, as the inoculation by trepanning with street rabies causes hydrophobia in a much shorter time than the interval of twenty-seven or twenty-eight days. I am, therefore, led to believe that they were sufficiently well inoculated to resist the bite of a rabid dog.

On the 28th August, 1886, two young dogs were inoculated beneath the abdominal skin, each with ten syringes of a medulla from the one hundred and twenty-second passage from rabbit to rabbit. These dogs did not suffer any apparent uneasiness during the following days, and to prove if they had become refractory to hydrophobia, they were inoculated, by trepanning, with a medulla from a rabbit inoculated with street rabies at the same time as a fresh rabbit, to try the virulence of the virus employed. The rabbit was taken with rabies the sixteenth day after trepanning, while the two dogs continued to do well the following months.

I could multiply infinitely these cases of immunity, as a consequence of subcutaneous inoculations with considerable quantities of different rabic virus. That in some cases hydrophobia does not result in consequence of these inoculations is surprising, on account of the quantity of virus inoculated, especially if one remembers that even the smallest fraction of this quantity of virus produces without fail hydrophobia, if the inoculation is made by trepanning. But what is especially surprising is, that in many cases, and without any apparent morbid phenomenon, an absolutely refractory state against the rabies is demonstrated. Can this latter effect not be understood more easily by the existence of a vaccine matter which accompanies the rabic microbes than by the action of the microbe itself? Without doubt this refractory state does not result in all cases, but one can understand that, for a variety of causes, the vaccine matter, if it exists, can not produce its effects under every circumstance, until the microbe lodges in a point favoring its culture. Moreover, without the existence of a vaccine matter, how can you understand the experience cited in the last instance, with two dogs inoculated beneath the skin, each with ten syringes of a very virulent matter from the one hundred and twenty-second passage from rabbit to rabbit, and who at first onset became refractory to the rabies? How the great quantity of rabic microbes, introduced beneath the skin, should not be cultivated here or there in the nervous system, if at the same time there was not introduced another matter, assimilating more quickly with this system, and placing the latter in a condition where it can no longer cultivate microbes? One can besides understand that also in the latter class of trials the experiment is not always successful, and that sometimes rabies will break out. Why, after all, in many circumstances should the rabic microbes not fix themselves in points where the nervous matter has not been preserved by the vaccine substance? One would naturally ask why the inoculation by trepanning should always produce rabies, and never a refractory condition. It would not be sufficient to answer that, by this manner of inoculation, the virus comes always and immediately in contact with the encephalon. To this argument might be objected, that many times an abundant inoculation beneath the skin might carry the virus and the elements by which it is formed to the encephalon, by means of the venous and lymphatic circulation, just as quickly and directly as by trepanning. The real difference between the two methods of inoculation seems to me to consist in the circumstance that the inoculation beneath the dura mater always introduced but a very trifling quantity of virus, and, in consequence of vaccine matter, which is not sufficient to produce a refractory state, while the quantities of the latter, introduced beneath the skin, are naturally much larger.

When a dog is bitten by a rabid dog, the bite does not always communicate the rabies; this is a well-proved fact. Such bites can introduce into the corporeal economy also only very small quantities of virus and preserving matter. Now, I have often tried if these dogs, bitten by rabid dogs, without having developed rabies in consequence, had become refractory to this malady, but in all cases, where I tried the inoculation by trepanning with rabic virus from street dogs, this operation gave them the rabies.

I have also made numerous trials to find out if, in the subcutaneous inoculations with rabic medullæ of successive passages from rabbits, the rabies would not be developed oftener by relatively smaller quantities of virus than by larger ones. I compared generally the effect of an inoculation with a quarter of a Pravaz syringe to that with one, two, or ten syringes. The result of these trials has often been: first, that rabies has seemingly developed more frequently after the application of a quarter of a syringe than after that of one or several syringes; second, that if the rabies did not appear, the employment of large quantities produced a refractory state oftener than that of small quantities.

One single experiment would be decisive to prove the presence of vaccine matter in the medullæ of rabbits which died from rabies. It would be necessary, if possible, to have in desiccation a series of medullæ which, by their inoculation on dogs, on jackals, or on rabbits, although deprived of virulence, would determine their refractory condition, because the microbe would lose its virulence before the vaccine matter could lose its preservative property.

In a great number of tests of this kind there are some, which have not enabled us to arrive at a conclusion fully devoid of uncertainty; some of the medullæ employed had retained a certain virulence. On other occasions the inoculations with those not retaining any virulence have not given the expected results, viz., the refractory state of the animals experimented upon. But on several occasions I have obtained some series of medullæ, of which not one grafted on rabbits by trepanning produced rabies, even after waiting for two or three months, and which, nevertheless, had produced the refractory state in dogs and jackals inoculated with them.

I have resumed the same experiments with other series of medullæ. Having failed in these trial tests, and finding myself diverted from my first favorable results, there arose in my mind serious doubts regarding the reliability of those experiments which I had considered conclusive, and I have resolved to take them up again as soon as I can find leisure. These are necessarily experiments of long duration, which ought to be repeated on the part of certain directors of anti-hydrophobic stations, who are in more favorable conditions regarding time at their disposal. The success of this kind of trials must consist in the use of medullæ, desiccated at a temperature as near as possible to that which kills all virulence in the rabic microbe. If medullæ, preserved in dry air at 25°, lose their virulence after an exposure of four or five days, these medullæ ought to be used, and even one ought to commence with medullæ the exposure of which has lasted six, seven, eight or more days.

It is unnecessary to describe the interest which the vaccination with or by means of non-virulent medullæ would offer. It would be not only a scientific fact of great importance, but also an invaluable progress in the method of preventing rabies.

To bring this letter, already too long, to a conclusion, I should like to speak on a last point of very great importance.

Certain facts, described in my note of 26th October, 1885, and the examples of inoculation of dogs, quoted in the present letter, give an idea of the important changes which take place in the conditions of rabic virus from street-dogs, when it passes to a first rabbit, and successively from rabbit to rabbit for a great many times. These changes can be charged to different causes. For example, the time of incubation of the rabies in the rabbits inoculated in succession may be considered. In the beginning the average of duration is fifteen days, when the virus of different rabid street dogs is inoculated in a first passage to rabbits. In this first passage, and from any street dog, I have never seen the time of incubation descend below eleven days, and even the duration of twelve and eleven days has been altogether exceptional. But by multiplying the successive passages, one descends to an incubating duration of eleven days; afterwards to ten and nine days, and later to eight days, where it remains for a long time, and finally towards the eightieth or one hundredth passage one has long since arrived at a duration of seven days, without ever recurring to eight days, even in exceptional cases. The duration of seven days continues for a very long time, descending only in exceptional cases to six days. To-day it still continues at seven days, after the one hundred and thirty-third passage from rabbit to rabbit. Can we believe that, in this respect at least, the rabic virus remains fixed? Will, by the always increasing number of passages, the time of incubation descend in a permanent manner to six days, at least for our breed of rabbits? Experience alone can decide these questions.

The further we remove from the original virus, and

from the virus of the first passages, the less susceptible becomes the hypodermic inoculation to determine the hydrophobia, especially with great quantities of virus, although giving place to a refractory state, as previously indicated by me.

It now only remains for me, my dear Duclaux, to speak of the duration of immunity, regarding the vaccinated dogs. You know, that at Villeneuve l'Etang I have been able to establish a vast kennel, where I have placed during two years a large number of dogs, rendered refractory to hydrophobia. At the end of the first year of their stay, I have tried on a group of their number, experimentally, the inoculation by trepanning with virus from street-rabies. The result was that eleven out of fourteen resisted. This year I have experimented on six other dogs, vaccinated two years since; four out of six have again resisted the inoculation by trepanning with virus from street-rabies, and one of the two, which took the infection, must have been partially vaccinated, as the malady did not break out till the twenty-eighth day after the trepanning. For the other, the twenty-first day was critical. And even these two might probably have suffered with impunity direct bites from rabid dogs. As regards the four refractory dogs, we know that the efficacy of preventive inoculation has been established.   L. PASTEUR.

(From the "Annales de l'Institut Pasteur" (book No. 1), by M. Duclaux.)

NOTE II.

"ON THE THEORY OF PREVENTIVE INOCULATION," BY M. A. CHAUVEAU.

. . . Until now the preventive inoculations known so far, as those of the small-pox, the cow-pox, the tag-sore or rot, the cattle peripneumonia, the splenic anthrax, the emphysematous carbuncle and the tetters, all had been made with the virus directly from the same maladies; strong, or more or less attenuated virus, the culture of which in the organism produces the outlines, or a rudimentary infection, of the source of immunity. But with the antirabic inoculations it is entirely different. Here it is no longer the virulent microbe which comes into play, but a special vaccine matter which accompanies it. Already Mr. Ferran pretended to bring about immunity by means of an anal-

ogous vacine matter, independent of the infectious agent.
Likewise Toussaint believed momentarily, that the carbunculous vaccination, which he obtained on sheep, in
his memorable experiment of 1880, with heated blood, was
due to a vaccine matter, dissolved in the inoculated blood.
But there the question was only of very problematic, and
even erroneous facts. The antirabic vaccinations of M.
Pasteur have for the first time shown, with the character of
a rigorous demonstration, the influence of a vaccine substance, entirely distinct from the pathogenic agent in the
creation of immunity. How can we connect this mode of
action, which seems to be entirely different, with that of
other preventive inoculations? . . . For this purpose we
will have to go back to the general mechanism of immunity, which necessarily blends with that of non-repeti-
tion.

The medical world has for a long time been divided in its
opinion about two theories: first, that of the absence or subtraction of the nutritive substances, which prepare the organism for the multiplication of infectious agents; second,
that of the presence or addition of detrimental substances,
opposed to this multiplication. M. Pasteur has accepted
the first theory, I the second. From the interpretation of a
very beautiful experiment of infectious culture "*in vitro*,"
M. Pasteur has drawn the foundations for his opinions.
Mine has been formed in consequence of a certain number
of facts, which the second theory alone can explain in the
pathogeny of infectious maladies.

Let us examine these facts.

I, as the first, have introduced into science the notion of
the influence which the number of infectious agents inoculated can exercise on the results of inoculation. Although at first hotly contested, this theory at present does
no longer meet with the same hostility as at the outset.
It even seems to me that M. Pasteur himself accepts it,
more or less explicitly; at least this is to be inferred from
his publication of the result of rabic inoculations with
medullæ in which the desiccation had destroyed more or
less numerous virulent elements.

In a communication of 28th June, 1880 ("Of the causes
which can change the results of carbunculous inoculations
on Algerine sheep. Influence of the quantity of infectious
agents. Application of the theory of immunity." By M.
A. CHAUVEAU. *Comptes rendus*, Vol. XC.), this influence
was first pointed out, as also the advantage derived there-

from, to explain the immunity. I demonstrate in the same by numerous experiments, that "the great quantity of infectious agents in the inoculation of splenic anthrax on Algerine sheep is one of the conditions which causes the defeat of the resistance which these animals generally offer to the carbunculous virus."

Further on I say: "A certain interest is attached to the facts exposed above, if they are considered under the point of view of their bearing on the trials of the general theory of immunity. . . . These facts . . . prove, that the carbunculous bacteridia behaves in the organism of Algerine sheep, not as if it were devoid of the necessary conditions for bacteridious life, but rather as if it were a medium which had been unfitted for that life through the presence of detrimental substances. In a very small number the bacteridiæ are prevented in their development by the inhibitory influence of those substances. In a very great number, on the other hand, they can surmount this obstacle to their prolification much more easily."

As this communication caused the intervention of M. Pasteur in vindication of the theory of exhaustion, I have taken up this interesting subject in another note (*Comptes rendus*, Vol. XCI., 18th Oct., 1880). . . . "By the way, I found a fact for the explication of which it would be difficult to apply the theory adopted by M. Pasteur, and I have stated it. This difficulty still exists. The question was the comparative study of inoculations executed, some with very small, others with very large quantities of infectious agents, on Algerine sheep, provided only with their natural immunity, as well as on those whose immunity had been strengthened by one or more preventive inoculations. I have demonstrated (and I am now able to make my demonstration still more complete) that there are many more chances of success to produce the splenic anthrax complete, that is to say mortal, with inoculations, introducing in the organism at a single stroke a great number of infectious agents. How can you make this fact agree with the theory of exhaustion? How can an organism from which have disappeared by means of one or more former cultures the greater part of substances necessary for the prolification of the infectious agents of carbuncle offer greater facilities for the pullulation of these agents with abundant seeds than with a quantity of seeds reduced to a minimum? If the poverty of the ground is an obstacle to the cultivation, ought not this cause of sterility manifest itself with as much stronger evidence, as this ground receives greater quantities of germs to be fecundated? What would certainly pass in a tube of cultivation, ought it not to show itself equally in the animal organism? This is my objection. I have formulated it in a theoretic interpretation of the facts observed, and said that "the bacteridic inoculations *comparatively with little or much virus* behave themselves in Algerine sheep *just as if the infectious agents* found in the organism of the animal *other substances* against which *the former had to contend*, so as to live and multiply, and which they could more easily overcome when they were in great number."

The confirmative facts did not fail soon to be multiplied. Under date of 4th April, 1881, in a special communication ("The Attenuation of the Effects of Virulent Inoculations by the Employment of very Small Quantities of Virus," by M. A. CHAUVEAU. *Comptes rendus*, Vol. XCII.) I confirmed the results of the preceding year by extending them to another virus, that of emphysematous carbuncle. It is therein proved: "That the quantity of virus employed for inoculating this malady exercises an enormous influence on the results of inoculations; the effect being always fatal when the quantity is very small." It is also proved: "That even in the highest degree of their benignity the effects of a first inoculation produce immunity."

Later the gangrenous septicæmia, which I studied in 1884 with Mr. Arloing, furnished still more demonstrative facts about the influence of the number of the virulent elements (*Bulletin of the Academy of Medicine*, of June and August, 1884). I shall not relate these facts in detail, as it will be sufficient to give the general significance of the same. This purpose will be filled by citing the following lines which I cull from the *Revue scientifique* (1885, Vol. II., page 619): "Probably by means of venous injections . . . the influence of the *number* of inoculated agents on the effects produced thereby, is demonstrated in the most remarkable manner. It has been proved . . . that the light sickness caused by these injections is very easily transformed into a serious, and even fatal infection, with exaggerated pullulation of virulent elements, when a great quantity of infectious germs is introduced into the blood." This citation applies more particularly to the gangrenous septicæmia. It is concluded by the following sentence, which has a much more general character: "A great number of attenuated virus inoculated on animals endowed with a great force of reception, or of strong virus inoculated on animals whose force of reception is feeble, behave in the same manner whatever may be the manner of inoculation chosen."

Naturally, as this demonstration of the influence of the number of virulent elements extended itself, it also extended the field of application of the theory which consists in attributing the immunity to the resistance caused doubtless by the presence of pernicious substances which prevent a prolification of the microbes.

The application of this theory on the acquired immunity arises, so to say, by itself. By multiplying, in case of natural maladies, or those acquired by preventive inoculations, these infectious agents remove perhaps from the organism, at least in certain cases, some substances needed for the constitution of the means of cultivation, which agree with these agents; but to prove this is very difficult. On the contrary, certain facts seem to establish that the principal cause of this acquired immunity and of a nonrepetition consists in the creation of a resistance, which is doubtless due to the pernicious substances deposited by the microbes of the first infection. In fact, these cases more than those of natural immunity have given me the means of proving that the resistance offered by the organism to the effects of another inoculation is often insufficient, if the latter is made with a very great quantity of infectious elements.

One of the most curious examples of the effects of very strong virus, introduced abundantly into an organism which has become ultra-refractory by means of repeated preventive inoculations, has been presented by an experiment which was related in *Comptes rendus* (Vol. XCI., 26th Oct., 1880), viz.: Eight sheep prepared by numerous previous inoculations of carbunculous virus have been used for this experiment. In none of them was it possible to produce even a slight uneasiness by new hypodermic injections of small quantities of virus. Then each received in the jugular an injection of from fifteen to seventy cubic centimetres of fresh carbunculous blood containing from twelve thousand to five hundred thousand millions of bacillæ. Only three of the sheep escaped the direct action of these bacillæ. One perished after sixteen hours from a general carbunculous infection which manifested itself in an over-acute manner, so to say, by a prodigious abundance of virulent agents in the blood and in the spleen. The other four had an infection localized in the cerebral *pia mater*, and died of bacillary meningo-encephalitis.

How can, in the matter of infection, this influence of the number of infectious agents be explained? Two theories offer themselves.

1st.—It can be supposed that all the virulent elements, of the same humor or the same cultivation, have not an entirely equal activity. Among them may perhaps be found some which are more energetic and capable of overcoming the resistance which destroys all the rest. Therefore, employing great quantities of infectious liquid for these inoculations, one augments the chances of introducing some of these rare, specially active, agents. This is the simplest explication.

2d.—Or also, supposing the uniform activity of all infectious microbes, from the same humor and of the same cultivation, to be demonstrated, one might admit, that the first manifestations of this activity, in the interior of the animal economy, consists in the secretion of a matter which carries the refractory organism back to the state of a medium favorable to the culture of microbes, by neutralization of the obstacle, which the first virulent evolution has left in its wake. In small number, the infectious agents secrete too little, to create around them such favorable atmosphere, which on the contrary happens easily if they are present in very great number. One might compare this first action of the infecting microbe, introduced into a refractory medium, to that of yeast in beer, which begins its work by the secretion of the inversive fermentation of Mr. Berthelot, which is the indispensable beginning for the exercise of the dividing action of the yeast on sugar.

Which is then this material, created in the virulent evolution, and which, by penetrating the elements of the organism, makes them unfit for a second evolution of the same nature?

Is it the ptomaine, this soluble poison, resulting from the microbic life and multiplication, a poison to which one must ascribe, as I have proved by the splenic anthrax, the greater part of the organic troubles and even death, in infectious diseases?

Is it something else? Nobody could tell. It is a result of the infectious evolution; that is all that is known: a result which by the more or less violent impregnation of the organism, puts the latter in condition to resist the work of every new infectious fermentation, as the alcohol, produced by the yeast in the first part of an operation, prevents by its accumulation, every new operation of division of sugar.

But if we do not know with which material we have to deal, we know at least one of its most important characters, that of its diffusibility in the organism. And this is one of the most interesting points in the acquired immunity.

The first indication of this character may be found in my study, under the title "Of the reinforcement of the immunity of Algerine sheep from splenic anthrax, by preventive inoculations. Influence of the mother on the receptiveness of the fœtus." (*Comptes rendus*, Vol. XCI., 19th July, 1880). I prove in the same, that pregnant ewes, inoculated with splenic anthrax, communicate to their offspring a remarkable increase of immunity, so that the lambs after their birth, offer a perfect resistance to carbunculous inoculations practised upon them.

"From this fact are derived important consequences for the theory of immunity, communicated or re-inforced by preventive inoculations. As M. Davaine has so lucidly demonstrated, the bacteridic spores are not multiplied in the blood of the fœtus, even if prodigious quantities are found in the mother's blood. Besides the normal solid elements of the blood do not commonly pass from one vascular system into another. The sanguineous plasma alone can give the object of active osmotic exchanges between the mother and the fœtus. We are therefore justified in our conclusions, regarding preventive inoculation of splenic anthrax: 1st, *that the direct contact of animal organism with bacteridic elements is not indispensable for the ulterior sterilization of that organism;* 2d, that preventive inoculations act on sterile and sterilizing humors, properly so called, either by the subtraction of substances, which are necessary for the bacteridian prolification, or *rather* by the addition of substances, which are pernicious to this prolification."

Since the publication of these lines, the question of the penetration of the bacillæ of carbunculous fever into the blood of the fœtus has made some progress, principally due to the intervention of Messrs. Strauss and Chamberland. "I could no longer say to-day, as I have done before, on the faith of Brauell and of Davaine, that the bacillæ of the mother's blood will not penetrate into the blood-vessels of the fœtus. There are certainly some cases, where the soluble poison is not alone the cause. It is moreover sufficient, that it should be sometimes found there (I speak here only of the ewe), for being authorized, to consider it as the agent of the intra-uterine immunity." I must repeat that: "I uphold the absolute exactitude of the facts, which establish this immunity. Those who wish to control them by realizing the conditions, which are necessary for their reproduction, and the conditions relative to the species of the mother, to the age of the fœtus, and to the number of inoculations, will never fail to observe what I have seen myself. Since the publication of my first facts, there never passes a year that I do not find occasion to practise in my laboratory repeatedly preventive inoculations on pregnant ewes, more or less near the end of their gestation. It is very rare that they drop prematurely. Nearly all arrive at their term, and give birth to healthy lambs which, at the age of four or six weeks, resist perfectly the inoculations of the strongest carbunculous virus." (*Revue scientifique*, 1884, Vol. II., p. 358.)

To sum up, these experiments have proved that the active matter in the production of immunity, can engender the latter in a medium, which derives this matter, by gradual osmotic diffusion, from another medium, the exclusive or nearly exclusive seat of production.

There is only a single step to the application of this theory to the case of two conjugate organisms. And really, I have thought that the carbunculous blood, deprived of its bacillæ, might communicate the immunity to other animals, *if one caused to pass by transfusion into the blood of the latter a great quantity, instead of the trifling doses which Toussaint wrongly believed capable of producing this result*. It is only in the *Revue scientifique* of 1884 (Vol. II., p. 358), that I have spoken of my experiments, which were all negative. I spoke in the following terms: "After the attempts, which I have made to communicate the anti-carbunculous immunity to sheep by the intra-venous injection of a great quantity of defibrinized blood, heated to a temperature capable of killing all the pathogenous bacillæ which it contains, this medium cannot at all be counted upon. It is true that the treatment which the infectious blood must undergo, does, perhaps, not alone act upon the vitality of the bacillæ, but even upon the essential quality of the poison, which we have reason to believe very alterable."

I have been obliged to cite this passage, so as to prove that my partial failure had not, in the main, shaken my

confidence in the scientific principle, which had inspired
my investigations. It is nevertheless certain that I have
not succeeded in producing immunity by the application
of this principle. The other attempts known at the time I
wrote the foregoing lines, had not been made under conditions favoring the belief, that the preservation, by means of
preventive inoculation, had ever been obtained otherwise,
than with really virulent substances, acting by means of
the infectious microbes which they contained. I was also
very little inclined to think that success could ever be obtained thus, when M. Pasteur published his second method
of anti-rabic inoculations.

With these anti-rabic inoculations a new era has been
opened. They give us the uncontestable proof of the vaccinal activity in the products of evolution of the virulent
agents. In the first liquids which were injected, these
agents existed no longer; they had all been killed by the
desiccation in the presence of air. These liquids are nevertheless active, because they prepare the organism for the
reception with impunity of new liquids, the injection of
which, at the first onset, and without preceding preparation of the organism, would provoke without fail mortal
rabies.

At the same time that they cap the theory of immunity,
these anti-rabic inoculations receive from this demonstration, or rather obtain for themselves, the scientific justification claimed by the partisans of this method. They do
no longer appear with the character of a peculiar exception,
but rather as a particular manner of making the vaccinal
matter active. In the ordinary preventive inoculations,
this vaccinal matter is gradually produced on the spot, by
the regular evolutions of the pathogenous microbes in the
very midst of the organisms of the inoculated subjects. In
the anti-rabic inoculations, the vaccinal matter produced
by another organism is put, already full formed, in contact with the subjects to be preserved first alone, and after-
ward accompanied by a gradually increasing number of
pathogenous agents; these latter, perhaps, also contribute
to produce the immunity, by being developed after the
manner of attenuated virus in a medium, prepared to favor only a rudimentary virulent evolution.

After all the preceding, the following propositions may
be established:

1st.—The immunity, acquired after a natural infectious
disease or after a preventive inoculation, may perhaps be

due in certain cases to the subtraction, by the first virulent evolution, of the proper material for the culture of the
specific microbe in the animal organism. But this immunity results especially from a resistance, brought about by
this first evolution, to a second evolution of the infectious
agent.

2d.—This resistance, in all probability, is the consequence
of the impregnation of the animal organism with a soluble and diffusible matter, either the specific poison, engendered by the multiplication of the pathogenous microbes,
or with any other substance resulting from the microbic
life, that is to say, of the infectious evolution.

3d.—It is not indispensable that this matter, in order to
produce a defensive effect against a new infection, or to
engender immunity, should be bred in the organism, as it
can fill this purpose merely by being provided with great
activity, and introduced into the economy in sufficient
quantity.

4th.—There is no essential difference between the preventive inoculation, practised after contamination and
that executed before. In both cases the object is to bring
about the immunity soon enough to prevent the infectious
evolution, which would follow the contamination if the
latter was left to its natural course.

5th.—The immunity communicated by the different
methods of preventive inoculations, is in reality acquired
by the same mechanism. There is no necessity of building up different theories for explaining the preventive
inoculation; all are blended in the general theory of immunity exposed heretofore.

Addition.—This note was already written when I was
made acquainted with the letter which forms, so to say,
the introduction to the *Annals of the Pasteur Institute.*
The second paragraph is entirely dedicated to this question:
" What idea can be formed of the cause of immunity by
means of the prophylactic method of rabies, after being
bitten ?" There is nothing in this letter which would not
agree with the developments just given by me, either according to M. Pasteur's ideas, or according to my own.
The theory of immunity acquired by the action of a proper
substance, dependent from the specific microbes, receives
even a fresh confirmation through some of the facts cited
in that letter; for example, those that show that there are
less chances of inoculating rabies, and more chances of

creating immunity by abundant injections of rabic liquid, provided with great virulent activity.

At first sight, these facts appear to be in contradiction to the numerous experiments by which I have demonstrated that the virulent elements of several infectious diseases have more influence in great than in small numbers, on more or less refractory organisms. But they only prove that in the case of rabies the vaccine matter which accompanies the infectious agents is very abundant, very energetic, and, above all, very quick in its action regarding these agents, while the reverse is the case for all the other diseases which have formed the subject of my investigation. (From the *Revue du Médecine*, Paris, 10th March, 1887.)

NOTE III.

On the first volume of the " Annals of the Institut Pasteur," and particularly on a memoir by Messrs. Roux and Chamberland entitled: "Immunity against the Septicemia conferred by Soluble Substances." Note by L. PASTEUR. (*Comptes rendus* of the Academy of Sciences, 30th Jan., 1888.)

The interesting memoir of Messrs. Roux and Chamberland demonstrates with perfect sharpness that the life of a septic vibrio develops soluble chemical products, which act gradually upon the former as if they were antiseptic. If they are introduced in sufficient quantity into the body of jackals, they confer upon the latter immunity against the mortal disease provoked by this vibrio.

Consequently it is proved that immunity against such a serious and rapidly mortal disease can be obtained by the injection of soluble and dosable chemical substances, and that these same substances are the result of the life of deadly microbes.

NOTE IV.

ON THE ELIMINATION BY THE URINE OF SOLUBLE, MOR-
  BIFIC, AND VACCINABLE MATTERS IN INFECTIOUS DIS-
  EASES, by M. BOUCHARD. (*Comptes rendus* of the Academy of Sciences, 4th June, 1887.)

. . . I am able to-day to establish, in regard to another infectious disease, the *pyocyanic malady*, that the urines of infected animals carry off, not alone soluble poisons

which are capable of reproducing in healthy animals some
of the symptoms of the infectious disease, but even the soluble vaccine matter which is capable of making the animals which are injected with these urines refractory to the
ulterior inoculation of the pathogenic organism. . . .

Animals previously injected with normal urine have not
acquired any immunity.

These experiments prove that the soluble, morbific, and
vaccinable matters can be produced by microbes in the
body of the affected animals the same as they are produced
in vitro, and that these soluble matters do not remain indefinitely in the body of the infected animals, and that they
are capable of being eliminated—partially, at least—by the
urinary secretion.

IMMUNITY THROUGH LEUCOMAINES.

This theory which, on account of its rationality and simplicity, presents the character belonging to truth, and which besides has in its favor the circumstances of being sustained by numerous experiments, realized in the laboratories of our scientists, might be qualified as a great discovery if, fortunately, it should be confirmed by the renewed experiments which it will naturally provoke. (*El Corresponsal de Paris*, 25th Sept., 1886.)

We are convinced that this interesting work will produce a lively impression in the scientific world on account of its novelty, and principally because it partly demolishes the bases until now accepted in micro-biological science. (*Europa y América*, Paris, Oct. 1st, 1886.)

This theory, whatever may be its final fate, which we cannot prejudge, is certainly one of those which best satisfy the spirit in the still very little known domain of the preserving causes, acting in the different prophylactic inoculations which are actually used. A hypothesis comes very near the truth when a whole class of phenomena finds thereby an explanation without shocking against a well-defined scientific principle. This is, according to all appearances, the case with the law laid down by Mr. B. . . . Although he is sufficiently modest to present it before the public only as a supposition, this supposition finds in the two organic reigns of nature so constant a confirmation that, until proof to the contrary be given, we may well consider it as a law of the creation.—P. DE BOUTAREL. (*Le Monde*, Paris, Oct. 4th, 1886.)

It is evident that the theory of the "Immunity through Leucomaïnes" seems to be confirmed by many facts, as, for example, that of alcoholic fermentation, detained by an addition of alcohol. It furnishes ingenious explanations for other facts. It can be found in the above-mentioned book. But as the author himself, who presents the defence of the same, recognizes, it has so far, like many others, only the character of a hypothesis.—ZABOROWSKI. (*La Justice*, Paris, 7 Oct., 1886.)

———

Mr. G. B. bases a complete theory on the employment of the leucomaines by means of inoculation nearly the same as it is practised by others, principally by M. Pasteur and the Spanish physician, Ferran, with bacteriæ or microbes. (*Le Mémorial Diplomatique*, Paris, 9th Oct., 1886.)

———

How does the vaccine act, and what is its origin? That is the question which Mr. E. G. B—— puts at the beginning of a work, which he has just published under the title of "Immunity through Leucomaïnes."

The author thinks he has found an answer to this question, and we believe that he may perhaps be right. . . . This theory is simple and seductive, and M. Pasteur seemed to have foreseen it when he said: "The rabic virus is accompanied by a non-virulent matter, which by itself is sufficient to determine the refractory state against the rabies." . . . Mr. E. G. B—— has done a thoroughly conscientious work. He has consulted all the authors—although they are very numerous—who have written about the infectious diseases, the microbes, the virus, etc., etc., and only after being convinced that all the facts, or nearly all, could be explained by his theory, has he presented the same to the public, persuaded that it would be recognized as true, and consequently might prove beneficial to humanity.—DR. H. VIGOUROUX. (*La Patrie*, Paris, 14th Oct., 1886.)

———

By the light of this theory the author examines successively all the great questions, which are yet litigious or obscure, and included in the great dogma of immunity, viz.: the principal prophylaxes, the return to virulence, the hereditary immunity, the attenuation of virus, etc. If we say that his different interpretations appear to be thoroughly reasonable, and that they give the key to a certain

number of morbid phenomena, hitherto unexplained, we
do him but justice. . . .

Nothing, assuredly, could be more interesting than these
probing strokes, delivered here and there into the depths of
the physiology of infinitely small bodies. The physician
and the naturalist are equally interested that these problems
should be agitated.—P. D. (*Lyon Médical*, official organ
of the "Société de Médecine" and of the "Société des
Sciences Médicales," 31st Oct., 1886.)

With the title of "Immunity through Leucomaïnes,"
there has been just published in Paris in French a very interesting work. It establishes with great distinctness and
solid argumentation a theory, as ingenious as simple,
which, if verified by the experiments which will certainly
follow in its wake, would reduce the multiple phenomena
of the infectious diseases to a natural and easily explained
law. (*La Dinastia*, Barcelona, 31st Oct., 1886.)

In the scientific circles of the capital of the neighboring
republic a very important work has been the subject of
frequent commentaries, and has been generally judged by
several scientific authorities of France with a very favorable criticism. (*El Barcelonés*, Barcelona, 1st Nov., 1886.)

. . . To call the attention of all friends of science to a
new theory of immunity, which is the object of the work
"Immunity through Leucomaïnes," recently published in
Paris by E. G. B., which by its merits has already been the
subject of favorable discussion in the press of the neighboring republic. The deductions which Mr. E. G. makes from
the principle admitted by him are so logical and are exposed with such conciseness and clearness of conception
that, if we follow him on the road which he travels with
sure steps over a rough and unexplored slope, we are sure
to arrive at the summit from where we discover an extensive horizon without limits. What we observe in the
foreground is real and positive; we can nearly touch it
with the hand without occasion for doubt. But what we
discover in the distance, will it be the same? It is necessary to arrive there. Let, therefore, the practical men, the
men of the laboratories, assist in the investigation and tell

us if the immense panorama of which the author of "Immunity" gives us a glimpse, is reality or only an illusion of mirage.—P. SANTALÓ. (*La Renaixensa*, Barcelona, 11th Nov. 1886.)

This theory is ingenious, the reasoning is simple, and ample justification of it is found in fact. If it be not exact, it is at least sufficiently plausible. (*The Morning Post*, London, 16th Nov., 1886.)

. . . Examining the pages of his book, one must admire the perfection which he reveals in having assimilated whatever has been written on the etiology and prophylaxis of infectious diseases.

Therefore science greets joyfully the author of this rational and simple theory for explaining the action of attenuated virus, which, should it receive the sanction of time or not, by all means will greatly assist those who devote themselves to the study of these arduous problems. (*Correo Catalan*, Barcelona, 15th Nov., 1886.)

. . . The book is entitled: "Immunity through Leucomaines" and in these brief words is contained, in a synthetical manner, the radical thought of the author's theory. In effect, the whole work is devoted to proving by experiments that all living beings, animal or vegetable, will find a principle opposed to its life in the leucomaines or alkaloids, produced by their vital functions; and he fortifies his demonstrations by a numerous series of curious facts.— M. VERDAGUER CALLIS. (*La Veu del Monserrat*, Vich, 20th November, 1886.)

. . . According to this we would no longer be in the presence of wonderful experimental results, like those of Jenner's vaccination or of the anti-rabic inoculations, of which results we cannot find the least serious explanation, but would be confronted by a theory and a method which would permit us to make, with a degree of certainty, unexpected discoveries in the so well surveyed, yet so little known, field of the infectious diseases. (*Revue du Monde Catholique*, Paris, 1st December, 1886.)

. . . He has looked over all authors—and to be sure they are very numerous—who have written on infectious diseases, and only after being convinced that all, or nearly all, their facts could be derived from the same principle, has he attempted, perhaps with too much timidity, to formulate a theory which he has submitted to the public in the expectation that it might be found true. . . . In the other parts of his work, Mr. E. G. B. gives the demonstration of his theory, and the explication by means of the same theory, of certain phenomena; there are especially some very curious chapters on the fermentation of wine and beer, to which we would call particular attention.—L. GRASI-LIER. (*Revue du Monde Latin*, Paris, 1st December, 1886.)

. . . As a consequence, the attenuation is nothing but the permanence of the microbe among the substances which it eliminates, and by which it is debilitated till perishing. In this form enter all the processes of elimination which the author of " Immunity through Leucomaïnes " explains with clearness and profound knowledge. That the microbes are accompanied by unassimilating substances has already been affirmed by Pasteur with regard to the virus of rabies, and by Ferran with regard to that of cholera.

Mr. E. G. B. has generalized these facts, by constructing the general law including them. (*La Publicidad*, Barcelona, 3d December, 1886.)

In the scientific circles of Spain, as well as of France, a book published lately by the firm of Berthier, successor of Leclerc, has caused much discussion. . . Mr. Güell's book will interest not alone those who are occupied professionally in these matters, but also those who, by their love of science and humanity, desire to keep posted about everything of importance regarding infectious and microbic diseases.—G. C. (*La Stampa*, Rome, 3d and 4th December, 1886.)

. . . We have passed over many arguments by which the author corroborates his theory, because they would lead us beyond the limits marked by the special nature of this publication; we only wish to say that those arguments, together with the general law in which they are founded, give good ground for the hope that Mr. E. G. B.'s theory will be confirmed by the ulterior discoveries of the men of science.—J. P. (*Industria é Invenciones*, Barcelona, 11th December, 1886.)

To sum up, as will be seen by the preceding notes, the work is extremely worthy of attention, on account of the judicious deductions which the author draws from the simplest facts, and shows an eminent spirit of observation, and if it leaves certain small blanks, as for example in reference to the natural immunity of some species against certain infectious diseases, they are of too little importance to destroy the essence of the theory. We fervently hope that new studies and experiments, which undoubtedly will be called forth by this work, will affirm the new path followed by the author, and will prove up to which point the observations transcribed by us are well founded.—JOSÉ M. BOFILL. (*La España Regional*, Barcelona, 12th December, 1886.)

"Immunity through Leucomaïnes," such is the theme studied by this scholar. It consists in introducing in the system, by artificial means, the leucomaines of the microbe, which produces the disease which one tries to prevent; in one word, it is to oppose the microbe by the microbe. Although we reserve our opinion, we must recognize that the question is treated with uncommon erudition. (*Le Petit Journal de la Santé*, Paris, 19th December, 1886.)

Whatever may be the outcome, the work of Mr. E. G. B. is the product of a conscientious seeker for truth; it requires a serious analysis, and we propose to make it, if you permit, on the occasion of our next discussion on the medicamental hypodermic injections.—President M. DANET, in the session of 7th October, of the Society of Practical Medicine of Paris. (*Revue Médicale*, for October, 1886.)

As we have seen, the theoretic concept of immunity is rational; but for the present we have still to deal with a hypothetic affirmation which requires further proofs of an experimental nature.

But neither must we forget that many of the modern triumphs of experimental nature have started from a simple hypothesis. Will that of Mr. Güell find some day the sanction of experiments? We hope it may be so, for the greater glory of science, and for the natural satisfaction of its author.—DR. ROBERT. (*Gaceta Médica Catalana*, Barcelona, 15th December, 1886.)

The author of this anonymous work proposes, with the most praiseworthy intentions, the difficult biologic problem: " How does the vaccine act, and which is its origin?" He constructs on this subject a very seductive theory, which permits him to explain the immunity by means of the leucomaïnes of the micro-organisms which, contained in the virus, would be opposed to its vitality.

Starting from this theory, Mr. E. G. B. draws from the same all possible conclusions, and endeavors to support his convictions by the successive study of chicken cholera, of anthrax, of hydrophobia, and of the fact, so interesting in micro-biology, of the return of virulence, of the hereditary immunity, and of the attenuation of virus.—DR. E. M. (*Journal de Hygiéne*, Paris, 16th December, 1886.)

It is undeniable that, notwithstanding the energetic and intelligent opposition of such eminent men as Peter, Collin, Gautier, Lefort, and many others whom we could name, the doctrine of microbes and the principle of preventive inoculation predominates in the field of medical science. But nevertheless it is certain that hitherto the relation which exists between one and the other, and therefore the manner of action of the second, has not been explained in a satisfactory manner.

The work whose title is given at the head of these lines has come to fill this gap; it is the production of an anonymous author, but whose competence and profound studies are revealed and confirmed in every one of its pages.—DR. MAÑE. (*Diario de Barcelona*, 18th December, 1886.)

Under the modest initials of E. G. B., there has been published in French a work which bears the title of " Immunity through Leucomaïnes," and, with the character of veritable actuality, unfolds an ingenious theory for explaining the immunity from infectious diseases by means of inoculations. . . . We can only recommend the reading of this book to all those who wish to inform themselves about the facts and the theory of immunity by means of preventive inoculation, as, besides explaining the theory of the author, it elucidates with perfect clearness and an abundance of detail the facts and experiments made regarding this subject.—P. M. (*Crónica Científica*, Barcelona, 25th December, 1886.

.... Supposing that you wish to treat of hydrophobia. What would you do? You will take a microbe, that is to say the venom which produces the disease, you cultivate it and you obtain a matter which preserves from this disease and annihilates it. What is this matter then? Evidently it is not a venom; it is not a thing which provokes the rabies; it is quite the opposite. But what is, it then? Mr. Güell, by means of the analysis and of the critics of the theories which exist on the subject, has arrived at a very simple and a very clear theory.—J. P. *Novoyé Vrémya* (New Times), St. Petersburg, 2d December, 20th November, 1886).

Under the title of "Immunity through Leucomaïnes, by E. G. B.," the publishing firm of Leclerc, successor to Berthier, in Paris, has published a very interesting work for micro-biologists, and of general utility, because it explains a principle, or rather a law of nature, which is very important for science.—DR. JUAN SANLLEHY. *El Criterio Médico*, Madrid, 31st December, 1886.

... In the absence of a satisfactory theory of the demonstrated preservative action of certain inoculations, this one is probably most easily sustained. (*Cosmos*, Paris, 20th December, 1886.)

The author has not made any experiments for the demonstration of his theory, but he makes admirable use of the discoveries of the last years, showing that he knows them thoroughly, and perhaps much better than any specialists, to present it as rational and verisimilar. In fact, he gives the whole history of what a certain famous German scientist would call the process of an hypothesis. And this really the contents of this interesting work are.—E. COROMINAS. (*El Barcelones*, Barcelona, 2d January, 1887.)

By all means, the theory of Mr. Güell is scientifically

true, and if the suppositions might be thought imaginary, the reasoning is not the less stringent and the conclusions not less logical.

Mr. Güell has thus indicated for the analysts a road, which can assist them materially in the study of comparative physiology, to give us a certain remedy for this disease, which prostrates by its sudden development, and strikes and appalls us by its mysterious propagation.—PROF. F. SABATINI. (*Roma Antologia*, Rome, 30th January, 1887.)

M. Pasteur has caused great progress in the vaccination in applying it to anthrax and hydrophobia; but how do these inoculations act ? This interesting question has remained until now unanswered. Mr. Güell y Bacigalupi has tried to lift the veil, which covers this mystery of pathologic physiology.

We naturally do not try to pronounce a judgment upon the value of this ingenious theory, based only on reasoning and not on experiments. But we do not hesitate in declaring that it has been unfolded with talent, erudition, and conscience. It only remains to add, that it is a very interesting reading. (*L'Italie*, Rome, 14th February, 1887.)

The anonymous author of this work has unfolded in the same a complete theory of immunity from contagious diseases, by means of vaccination, by supposing that the leucomaïnes of a pathogenous microbe are a poison for the microbe itself, and it is due to the persistent influence of these leucomaines, that the microbic diseases are unable to develop.

The vaccination only acts as a means of introducing in the organism the leucomaïnes of the microbes, which precede the disease, which one desires to prevent. (*Paris Médical*, Paris, 15th Feb., 1887).

"Immunity through Leucomaïnes," this is the title of a noteworthy book, recently published in Paris by Mr. E. G. B., and which is the object of heated polemics in the scientific world. . . . Pasteur and Ferran have demonstrated that the microbes are accompanied by disassimilated matter, and Mr. E. G. B. has generalized the demonstration of the facts, and formulated the law, which governs them. (*El Correo*, Madrid, 24th Feb., 1887.)

The author of this pamphlet believes that the immunity from any infectious disease, obtained by means of vaccination, is produced by the action of leucomaïnes, secreted by the microbes, which are inoculated in the vaccination. He says that this is the effect of a general law, as the substances produced and eliminated by all organic beings are poisonous for these same beings. The author defends his thesis by means of ingenious arguments, and his work is very interesting reading. (*Revue de Médecine*, Paris, 10th Feb., 1887.)

. . . By what we have said above, our readers will understand the importance of Mr. Güell's work, as it treats of a point of much interest for medicine, which regards not alone immunity in itself, but also is in intimate relation to the great problem of vaccination, and others of not less importance, as for example the cause of the spontaneous termination of infectious diseases, and the advantages or difculties resulting from either active, or on the contrary only symptomatical therapeutics.

Mr. Güell has explained the question of immunity with excellent judgment, formulating a new theory, which actually explains the immunity in a more scientific manner, and if in some details, as that of the law of habit in poison, we cannot fully agree with him, in all essential points we are of the same opinion as he.—CARRERAS, SOLA. Communication from Davos Platz (Switzerland) of 15th Jan., 1887. (*Revista de Ciencias Médicas*, Barcelona, 10th Feb., 1887).

It is evident that the theory of "Immunity through Leucomaïnes" seems to be confirmed by many facts, such as the alcoholic fermentation, suspended by the addition of alcohol. It furnishes ingenious explications of other facts, as can be seen from the book which we announce. (*Le Moniteur de Rome*, 31st Dec., 1886.)

The author passes in review the different virulent diseases, the microbes of which we know, and shows in what manner they confirm his theory. We cannot follow him through his extended development of the vaccine of chicken cholera; the carbunculous vaccination; the prophylaxis of rabies; the return of virulence; the hereditary immunity; the crisis of infectious diseases; the law of getting accustomed to poisons, etc.—JULLIEN. (*Revue des Sciences Médicales*, Paris, 15th Jan., 1887.)

"Immunity through Leucomaïnes" is the title of a book, the author of which is Mr. Güell.

The doctrine of microbes, and the principal preventive inoculations which in the latter years have given rise to so many controversies, and so many hypotheses, are unfolded with great erudition and great clearness by our intelligent author.

The theory of Mr. Güell is founded on the following principle: Every animated being produces substances, poisonous for its proper life. However, the leucomaïnes produced by a being, at the same time that they are poisonous for the same being, are inoffensive for other beings.

This theory is strengthened by the author with several experiments, by means of which satisfactory results are obtained on contagious diseases. (*Igea*, Rome, 6th Feb., 1887.

In running over the pages of this book, in one volume octavo, we must admire the perfection with which the author has assimilated whatever has been written in regard to the etiology and prophylaxis of contagious diseases.

The author strengthens this theory with a great number of experiments, by which he easily unfolds many phenomena peculiar to contagious diseases.

Science gratefully salutes the author of this rational and simple theory, which will render great service to all who dedicate themselves to the study of these arduous problems. —(*L'Osservatore Romano*, 10th Feb., 1887.)

The author adduces many proofs to strengthen his theory, which, to say the least, is ingenious. We refer the reader to the pamphlet itself, if he wishes to examine the question thoroughly. (*L'Univers*, Paris, 7th March, 1887.)

. . . This work is devoted to the experimental demonstration, that every living being, animal or vegetable, will find a principle opposed to its life in the leucomaïnes, or alkaloids, produced by its own vital functions; and this thesis is strengthened by a multitude of very curious facts worthy of being studied. Therefore, it is not strange that a work of this special character should have attracted attention at home and abroad, as not alone medical science will be directly benefited, but also agriculture in all its branches, especially as regards the diseases of cattle and plants, as also several rural industries. The studies made by M. Pasteur respecting the silkworm, sheep, swine, oxen, etc., fully prove the importance of this work, as the curative principles of these and other diseases are founded on the theory explained according to his criterion by the author of "Immunity by Leucomaïnes."—F. (*L'Art del Pagés*, Barcelona, 9th April, 1887.)

. . . The author strengthens his theory with an abundance of bibliographic documents; he finds in the works of Pasteur, Chauveau, Ferran, and others, arguments to justify his thesis. (*Le Progrés Médical*, Paris, 23d April, 1887.)

In the work of which we treat can be found beautiful theories, founded on plausible hypotheses; it cites numerous facts and observations, in the discussion of which the most eminent scientists have taken part; it relates experiments of Pasteur, and of our countryman Ferran, of the veterinary surgeons Bouley and Chauveau, members of the Academy of Sciences, and of other notabilities, whose concurrence increases the value of the work which we review. (*Diario de Zaragoza*, 3d June, 1887.)

The work in which Mr. G—— has explained his ideas was printed some months ago in Paris, under the title of "Immunity through Leucomaïnes." It is an exact, clear, and methodical recapitulation of the acquisitions of contemporaneous science in France and foreign countries, regarding this important subject. I can only recommend the perusal of the same to every one who wishes to keep up with all the latest attempts to counteract the greatest scourges of humanity, typhoid fever, yellow fever, hydrophobia, and cholera. The careful investigator will find in the same great advantage and economy of time spent in often difficult researches, and a statement of conclusions, which will recommend themselves to every unprejudiced mind.

At the moment of writing this review, the *Revue de Mé-*

décine brings me a very well written essay of Professor Chauveau of Lyons, on preventive inoculations for virulent diseases. His conclusions are identical with those of our author. I take special pleasure in calling the attention of physicians to this concordance between two scientists, unknown to each other, and separated by distance as well as by nature of their respective works.—M. DE NANT. (*L'Avenir de Lot et Garonne*, Nimes, 29th June, 1887.)

. . . This is the title of an important book published in Paris by the firm of Louis Leclerc, the anonymous author of which only signs with his initials. He treats his subject with a large amount of knowledge and penetrating judgment, putting his theory in close relation with the facts recently discovered regarding the pathogeny of virulent diseases, and the immunity to be obtained by special preventive vaccinations, and showing himself fully competent to wrestle with so difficult a material. . . .

The author shows much subtlety of intellect in adapting in favor of his theory the facts published by the ablest experimentalists. Without any prejudices for the future of his theory, we only wish to say that it seems worthy to be taken into consideration, and to be submitted to trial.—P. (*L'Imparziale*, Messina, 22d July, 1887.)

Really we must confess that on perusal of this book we were unable to leave it until we had entirely finished the contents. The manner of expressing the ideas seems extremely clear, the theory is demonstrated by experiments of the most distinguished microbiologists, and where they are wanting, the author calls to his assistance the most rigorous logics. (*Revista de Laringologia, Otologia y Rinologia*, Barcelona, 1887.)

A very important conclusion is established by this theory; in fact, if the leucomaïnes prevent the development of microbes, by which they are produced (and are therefore the veritable cause of the immunity), the preventive vaccinations must consist in the introduction of leucomaïnes peculiar to those microbes, the disease of which shall be prevented. This theory, expounded by Mr. Güell y Bacigalupi with clear logic and highly scientific reasoning, is worthy of study and observation, being specially adapted for them by the facts on which it is founded, and besides, it tries to solve a problem the importance and interest of which everybody must recognize.

We must confess frankly, that this theory strikes us as very ingenious; therefore, we add our humble but sincere expression of admiration to those which the author of "Immunity through Leucomaines" has already received from the medical profession.—Dr. FARRIOLS ANGLADA. (*Boletin de Medicina y Farmacia*, 28th Aug., 1887.)

. . . The theory of the author of "Immunity through Leucomaïnes" has such a character of universality, and rests so firmly on a law which already nobody can doubt, that it will be extremely difficult to demonstrate the opposite of what he asserts, and by all means he has opened the way, by his theory, for investigating the exact prophylactic action of vaccine.—AUGUST PI GIBERT. (*La Illustració Catalana.*)

Mr. Güell Bacigalupi has published a monograph ("Immunity through Leucomaïnes," Paris, 1886,) in which, with an abundance of data, he explains by means of a new theory the immunity which an individual who has been inoculated, or suffered certain diseases, enjoys for a certain time. . . . We frankly confess that this theory pleases us. (*Los Avisos Sanitarios*, Madrid, 20th Sept., 1887.)

Under the modest disguise of his initials, with which our countryman, Mr. Güell, signs his precious book, which forms a volume in octavo of 164 pages, that gentleman gives us a compendium of the actual knowledge regarding leucomaines, expounds the theory of immunity, gives the demonstration of this theory, and explains by the same certain phenomena.

We will later give further details on this book. (*La Medicina Castellana*, Valladolid, 27th Feb., 1887.)

Does immunity exist? And how can we acquire it? That in two words is the question which the author puts. It is expounded with great care, showing that the author has a great habit of observation. This book is full of information, and has the merit of being in accordance with the present state of an arduous question; and if the theory

accepted by the author does not satisfy every reader, he
will at least find under an agreeable and easy form the
consolatory hope which humanity may entertain should
the hypothesis be confirmed by experience.—DR. ROORYCK.
(*Journal de Médécine de Paris*, 13th Nov., 1887.)

As may be seen, the tendency of this work is to explain
the great and difficult problem of immunity which, in the
actual state of science, is still an enigma, as man himself
who is the object of same.   The reasoning is very ingenious, and is fortified by authoritative testimony; it is not
the less true that immunity is certain in the majority of
cases, either acquired by preventive inoculations or hereditary.   But the actual state of our knowledge does not
permit us to decide if the theory of M. Pasteur is to be
blamed, or if the prophylactic property of the leucomaines
must be recognized.   We can close this report by recalling
our sentence at the opening of this analysis.   This work,
product of experimentation, seeks to shed light on the
difficult question of micro-organism.   We can only en-
courage the seekers after truth to follow this new path,
which perhaps may lead them to the veritable pathogeny.
The work is worthy of being read, even if its perusal only
gives the reader the consolatory hope that immunity for
contagious diseases may be found.   (*Bulletin de la Société
d'Ethographie*, No. 11, Paris, 1887.)

www.ingramcontent.com/pod-product-compliance
Lightning Source LLC
Chambersburg PA
CBHW021803190326
41518CB00007B/430